PSYCHIATRY FOR SOCIAL WORKERS

PSYCHIATRY
FOR SOCIAL WORKERS

BY

ALISTAIR MUNRO, M.D., M.R.C.P.E., D.P.M.

Senior Lecturer and First Assistant,
Department of Psychiatry, University of Birmingham,
Honorary Consultant in Psychiatry to the Queen Elizabeth Hospital, Birmingham,
and to Birmingham Regional Hospital Board

AND

WALLACE McCULLOCH, M.Sc., A.A.P.S.W., M.R.S.H.,

Senior Lecturer in the Schools of Studies in Applied Social Studies,
University of Bradford

THE QUEEN'S AWARD
TO INDUSTRY 1966

PERGAMON PRESS

OXFORD · LONDON · EDINBURGH · NEW YORK
TORONTO · SYDNEY · PARIS · BRAUNSCHWEIG

Pergamon Press Ltd., Headington Hill Hall, Oxford
4 & 5 Fitzroy Square, London W.1
Pergamon Press (Scotland) Ltd., 2 & 3 Teviot Place, Edinburgh 1
Pergamon Press Inc., Maxwell House, Fairview Park, Elmsford,
New York, 10523
Pergamon of Canada Ltd., 207 Queen's Quay West, Toronto 1
Pergamon Press (Aust.) Pty. Ltd., 19a Boundary Street,
Rushcutters Bay, N.S.W. 2011, Australia
Pergamon Press S.A.R.L., 24 rue des Écoles, Paris 5e
Vieweg & Sohn GmbH, Burgplatz 1, Braunschweig

Printed in Great Britain by The Anchor Press Ltd., Tiptree, Essex

Contents

Contents

Contents

Foreword

ONE of the features of modern psychiatry is the growing number of different kinds of professional workers who are likely to become involved with it. While mental illness is primarily a medical affair, the problems which it presents are so extensive that the psychiatrist needs all the help he can get from colleagues in other relevant professions. Psychiatrists cannot work in isolation any more than surgeons, unless of course only very minor operations are envisaged. A psychiatric and a surgical team have in common the need for co-operative effort on the part of those who constitute it. But if a team is to function effectively there are certain prerequisites. Each team member must know what his function is in relation to his colleagues. This of course cannot be achieved merely by agreement. A specialist role demands specialist training though based on a common body of knowledge presented in a form most useful in relation to the particular specialist role envisaged. This is why this book came to be written.

The literature of psychiatry is enormous and grows larger every day. And yet by no means all those who have recourse to it have their needs adequately catered for. It is inevitable that psychiatrists themselves come off best. The needs of medical students and non-psychiatric physicians are now almost as well met. This book, however, is for social workers and is directed specifically at them. Appropriately it is a joint effort. One of its authors is a psychiatrist, the other a former psychiatric social worker and now a lecturer in applied social studies.

In writing such a book it is vital to achieve a balance. In the face of uncertainty, there is an understandable tendency towards a too ready acceptance of a body of knowledge which is all too easily translated from the realm of hypothesis to which it quite properly belongs to the realm of fact where it quite improperly belongs. But such an acceptance of non-facts as facts does no more than produce an illusion of certainty. One method of counterbalance is the provision of a sound text. In view of this, this book should fulfil a real need.

W. H. TRETHOWAN

Professor of Psychiatry,
Dean of the Medical Faculty,
University of Birmingham

Editor's Foreword

PROFESSOR TRETHOWAN is right to emphasise the team approach in the recognition and treatment of psychiatric illness, but we should not necessarily think of this team as being within the four walls of a hospital. Psychiatry is showing a healthy tendency to emerge from hospital into the community and in doing so it leans much more heavily than before on the assistance of every type of social worker. It is important that disciplines which have previously been separated by the high wall of the mental hospital should now learn to communicate with each other. This book has been written for all workers in the social work field with the purpose of facilitating this type of communication where it affects people who are mentally ill either by collaborating in their treatment or by bringing help to them when their illness has not previously been recognised. It will be especially useful for social work students.

University of Bradford   JEAN P. NURSTEN

Introduction

THIS is not a comprehensive text-book of psychiatry. There are many of these already available, but since they are written *for* psychiatrists *by* psychiatrists they make heavy reading for the layman and so far as the social worker is concerned they contain far too much specialized information about matters like diagnostic procedure and details of treatment.

In the course of their profession, social workers in all fields are bound to come in frequent contact with situations where a psychiatric problem is an important factor and so they must have an adequate working knowledge of psychiatry. They should be able to recognize psychological illness for what it is and should be able to communicate their observations to their colleagues. When they are involved in the social or therapeutic aspects of a psychiatric case they should appreciate the significance of their own contribution. The social worker must have an intelligent interest in psychiatry but this does not necessarily imply that he or she must have an exhaustive knowledge of the subject.

We have tried to give a well-balanced and non-sectarian view of psychiatry and we have stressed those aspects which are of especial interest or importance to the social worker. We have deliberately excluded the topics of child psychiatry and mental subnormality because we believe that these require separate treatment, but otherwise we have endeavoured to give a general view of present-day psychiatry. This book is detailed enough to serve the trainee social worker for examination purposes and the trained worker for professional purposes, but we hope that its presentation of psychiatry is sufficiently interesting to encourage the reader to seek further knowledge in more specialized texts.

On pp. 272ff. of this volume will be found a list of books which we recommend for this purpose.

Acknowledgements

WE WISH to extend our especial thanks to Mrs. Rita Richardson of Messrs. Roche Products Ltd. who prepared the bulk of our manuscript. We would also like to thank Mrs. A. Sugden and Mrs. V. McGuinness, Secretaries, Schools of Studies in Applied Social Studies, University of Bradford, and Miss C. Davies, Secretary, University of Birmingham, for their considerable help. Mrs. Valerie Freeman gave valuable assistance in preparing the index.

We must mention with gratitude our wives and families who never grumbled while undergoing the considerable degree of paternal deprivation which spare-time authorship involves.

CHAPTER 1

Introducing Psychiatry

The Historical Background to Present-day Psychiatry

Mental illness occurs in all human societies and so far as we can tell has always done so. Throughout the ages the mentally ill have been treated at different times with awe, contempt, rough humour or with savage persecution. Nowadays mental illness no longer produces the same feeling of dread that it once did, but it has taken a long time for the stigma attached to it to begin to disappear. (Tuberculosis once carried the same sort of stigma, but in recent years the prevention and treatment of this illness have become so efficient that the fear it used to generate has almost vanished: the same process is now occurring in psychiatry.)

To their credit the Ancient Greeks recognized that mental illness was indeed a form of sickness and that it required treatment based on reason and not on superstition. Their views regarding the causes of these illnesses were naïve, but their insight was commendable. Unfortunately their example was rarely copied in later times and the subject was once more plunged into an atmosphere of unreason. The spread of Christianity into Europe had the incidental result of introducing the Jewish belief that insanity was due to possession by evil spirits and this became incorporated in Christian thinking. During the Middle Ages and even later many of the insane were persecuted as witches. Those who were not regarded as agents of Satan were consigned to mad-houses whose main purpose was to keep the inmates out of the sight of polite society (except when it became fashionable for the members of society to visit these institutions for amusement, paying a fee to watch the lunatics much as nowadays we go to look at the animals in the Zoo). Treatment was ineffective and the emphasis was almost entirely on custody. Because of this, most people with mental illness only entered hospital when their condition was so advanced that they could no longer be tolerated in society. If recovery occurred it was usually due to a natural remission of the illness rather than to treatment: many poor wretches did not recover and they dragged out the rest of their lives in confinement and not infrequently in chains.

With a few humane exceptions this was the position until the latter part of the eighteenth century. Medical science had made many advances since the beginning of the previous century, but it took a full hundred and fifty years for more enlightened views on the nature of mental illness to begin to prevail. By the end of the eighteenth century the mentally ill were being released from their shackles and during the following hundred years many new mental hospitals were built in Britain, the United States and Europe. They were founded in a spirit of enlightenment and a much more hopeful attitude developed towards the treatment of psychiatric illnesses although the treatments themselves were still relatively ineffective.

Nowadays when we look around we can see the legacy that the psychiatry of last century has left us. This has mostly taken the form of large mental institutions, often forbidding in appearance and in many cases built in remote and inaccessible places so that the patients could not be a nuisance to the community. There was still a heavy emphasis on custody and a high proportion of the people who were admitted to hospital remained chronic inmates. Because of their illness many psychiatric patients show an extreme tendency to withdraw into themselves and before long they become institutionalized: this can usually be prevented nowadays, but previously it used to happen a great deal and when it did the prospects of discharge became remote. After a time relatives and friends would die, disappear or ignore the patient, who then became utterly isolated from general society. Apathetic and withdrawn, he led an almost vegetable-like existence. Despite these circumstances little attention was paid to the need for active social work. If a patient's relatives became destitute as a result of his prolonged incarceration they might receive charity of some sort. Social workers, such few as there were, were almoners in the old sense of the word, dispensing alms to the needy. Usually a strong moral attitude was taken with the relatives, who were expected to shift for themselves, and there was little thought of a preventive approach or of active case-work with the patient or his family.

In order to put the treatment of mental illness on a more logical basis an improved method of classifying the various conditions was needed. During the second half of the nineteenth century a number of French psychiatrists made important contributions in this direction: thereafter the initiative passed largely to German psychiatry which laid down the basis for much of our present-day classificatory system. In particular, Emil Kraepelin (1855–1926) is regarded as having taken the outstanding part in this work. He laid great stress on the need for careful observation of many patients over long periods of time in order to be able to draw general conclusions about the illnesses from which they suffered.

Kraepelin's work was especially valuable for the light it threw on the psychotic illnesses. These are the most severe forms of mental illness and are the ones which lay people associate with the concept of "insanity". Nowadays a great deal of psychiatric practice is concerned with another group of conditions, the psychoneuroses. Conventionally these are regarded as less severe forms of psychiatric illness though, in fact, they often cause a great deal of distress to the patient and his family. Until nearly the end of the nineteenth century there was a tendency to regard the psychoneuroses not as illnesses at all but as signs of moral or constitutional weakness. Most people considered the manifestations of mental illness to be gross disturbances of thinking or behaviour. Individuals who were tense or afraid or unhappy, but nevertheless rational, were not "mad" so they were not usually considered to be ill.

This viewpoint was beginning to change in some quarters, but the change was given enormous impetus by the work of Sigmund Freud (1856–1939) and his associates. They drew attention to the frequent occurrence of emotional disorders and showed that individuals suffering from such disorders, though far from insane, could still be intensely unwell and deserved treatment every bit as much

3

as the patients with psychoses. As well as this Freud devised a system of psychology which attempted to show how the psychoneuroses develop. He also devised a method of treatment which was derived from his psychoanalytic theories. Psychoanalysis and its various offshoots have had an enormous influence, not only in psychiatry but in society generally. Nowadays many of its theoretical assumptions are being challenged and its efficacy as a form of treatment is seen to be considerably more limited than was once thought, but in the early part of the present century it engendered a great deal of therapeutic optimism and intellectual curiosity which greatly benefited psychiatry. As well as this, psychoanalysis stressed the need to consider each individual's problems in depth; this meant that the thoughts and feelings which went on within the patient developed significance for diagnosis and treatment. This inevitably involved the consideration of factors, such as work, the family, interpersonal relationships, the individual's adequacy to cope with everyday problems and so on. As a result the emphasis has moved away from the chronic patient who was isolated in an institutional setting and nowadays is much more concentrated on the individual in his social milieu. Interest in the significance of social factors in psychiatric illness has greatly increased and the need for the modern type of social work has developed accordingly.

Psychiatric theory and the classification of mental disorder have made great advances in the past hundred years, but until comparatively recently the efficacy of treatment failed to keep pace. With the development of psychoanalysis some neurotic conditions could be cured and many could be alleviated, but until the 1930's many psychiatric illnesses remained resistant to the treatments which were available. There was one exception to this: at the time of the First World War it had become possible to treat general paralysis of the insane which used to be an extremely common form of dementing illness and which was due to brain-damage brought about by the organism causing syphilis. It had been noted that sometimes a severe feverish illness with high temperature could have the incidental effect of destroying the syphilitic organism, with consequent improvement of the mental illness. Patients were therefore deliberately infected with malaria which produced severe fever and when this had cured the cerebral infection the malaria was then treated. The treatment was drastic but often effective: afterwards drugs were developed which directly attacked the infection and with the appearance of penicillin general paralysis of the insane (G.P.I.) virtually vanished.

The effectiveness of this treatment in a particular psychotic illness was very heartening to psychiatrists because it encouraged them to believe that other hitherto untreatable psychoses could perhaps be successfully dealt with. However, few dramatic advances occurred until almost the end of the 1930's. Certainly new and more effective sedative drugs had appeared and with these it was possible to control disturbed behaviour more efficiently, but they did not actually affect the illness itself. Anticonvulsant drugs became more sophisticated at about the same time and it was therefore possible to treat epilepsy much more satisfactorily.

Just before the Second World War, two important treatments came into use. The first was used in the therapy of schizophrenia and consisted of the inducing of a series of comas in the patient by means of large doses of insulin. This treatment is no longer used because more effective drugs have become available, but for twenty years it was the mainstay of the treatment of schizophrenic illness. At about the same time as insulin coma treatment was introduced it was observed that artificially induced seizures could relieve severe depression, so for a time drugs which produced generalized fits were used to treat this illness. This often removed the depression, but their side-effects could be unpleasant and dangerous, so they were superseded by electroconvulsive therapy (E.C.T.). This latter form of treatment essentially consists of passing an electric current through the brain and is usually extremely effective in removing depressive symptoms. Originally it was a somewhat unpleasant procedure which, as a side-effect, produced a convulsion, but now, in its much safer and modified form, it is combined with drugs which prevent convulsions yet do not prevent the beneficial effects.

Depressive illness is usually self-limiting—that is, it will tend to cure itself after a time if no complications (such as suicide) occur. E.C.T. does no more than hasten recovery, but since it used to be fairly common for an attack of depression to last up to several years at a time (though the majority were very much briefer than this), obviously such a treatment was important since it would enable a depressive patient to recover from his condition in the foreseeable future. With the advent of E.C.T. for depression and insulin coma treatment for schizophrenia the stigma attached to mental illness really began to recede because it was realized that these severe and mysterious diseases were at last accessible to therapy. Mental hospitals now became treatment centres instead of detention centres: it started to be "respectable" to have a psychiatric illness and the use of outpatient treatments became feasible.

Unfortunately many mental hospitals are situated in inconvenient places, to a great extent cut off from the community at large. In recent years there has been a growing emphasis on the need to keep patients in touch with the community, their homes and family. For this purpose, outpatient treatment is obviously preferable but many patients still need to come into hospital. In order to reduce separation from their normal environment to the minimum the modern trend has been to open psychiatric units in general hospitals: these are often more conveniently situated and there is usually relatively little resistance on the part of the patient to being admitted there. Mental hospitals still carry out a very large proportion of psychiatric work (including nowadays the growing problem of the long-term care of the mentally deteriorated elderly patient), but psychiatric departments in general hospitals have played an important role in rendering psychiatric treatment more acceptable and more convenient.

All of this has been made infinitely easier by the introduction during the 1950's of a number of tranquillizing drugs of different types. Some of these have proved effective in the treatment of schizophrenia and have replaced insulin coma treatment. Others can lessen severe anxiety or control disturbed behaviour. All of them have made it much more possible for the severely ill psychiatric patient to be treated in a non-psychiatric hospital and have made him accessible to forms of psychotherapy which previously could not have helped him. They have also accelerated the discharge of many patients from hospitals and have enabled large numbers to be treated in day hospitals or as outpatients. An incidental benefit of all this has been that workers in the psychiatric field no longer need to work separately from society: since many patients remain in the community or at least keep close ties with it, psychiatric staff have been able to reduce their degree of professional isolation.

Nowadays there is a desire to seek new and ever more effective treatments, whether these be psychological or physical. There is every incentive to catch the illness at an early stage to prevent its reaching a severe and intractable form. It is now realized that hospital psychiatry is only "the tip of the iceberg" and that the great majority of milder psychiatric disorders in the population either go unrecognized or are dealt with by the general practitioner. There is a growing interest in the psychiatric problems which can aggravate physical disease, produce problem families, result in inefficiency and absenteeism from work, etc., and community psychiatry is getting under way. Of course, we all hope that the ideal of preventive psychiatry will some day be achieved: to catch the potential patient and prevent his illness before he ever needs to come near hospital. This largely remains an unrealized aim, but we are certainly seeing the patient much sooner than once was the case and if he does have to enter hospital we are acutely aware that he must not be allowed to become institutionalized and that his relatives must not be allowed to develop a way of life which excludes him. All of these trends demand more and more in the way of active social work alongside the psychiatric treatment.

The Role of Social Work in Present-day Psychiatry

Psychiatrists are medical practitioners whose training enables them to recognize the signs and symptoms of mental disorder. When the psychiatrist has decided on the diagnosis his main concern is to help the patient to get better as soon as possible with the minimum of suffering. In order to effect a cure he has to apply the most appropriate form of treatment: in comparison with other branches of medicine psychiatric treatment is still very empirical, but the degree of specificity with which therapy can be prescribed is increasing all the time.

A doctor's life is spent in the recognition and treatment of disease and it is often said with some justification that he is more interested in the illness than in the person who is ill. He is often so busy trying to cure the patient that at times he almost ignores the human factor. Of all medical specialists, psychiatrists must be the most aware that any illness is inextricably intertwined with the sufferer's total personality: the personality may affect the appearance of the illness and the illness may in turn affect personality and behaviour. This may also produce alterations in the behaviour of other family members, resulting in their estrangement from the patient and consequently further deterioration of his mental state. Treatment, to be wholly effective, must take into account the "whole person", and when we are dealing with a psychiatric illness we must be aware of the many factors which may be of importance in the illness though not necessarily part of it. Often these factors are of social significance: for example, it is not easy to treat a depressive illness when the man suffering from it is constantly worried that he may lose his employment. Nor is it likely that drugs will cure an anxiety state in a woman if the fact is overlooked that she is destitute because her husband has deserted her and has left her to look after a large family of children.

It is the psychiatrist's duty to treat mental illness as effectively as possible. Sometimes he may be able to tackle the social problems which contribute to his patient's anxieties, but he rarely has time to become deeply involved in this aspect. In order to gain the patient's confidence and to maintain a therapeutic relationship it is often valuable to have someone else who deals with the family and copes with environmental problems. And, if the truth be told, the psychiatrist is often less skilled in dealing with the social aspects of the problem than the experienced case-worker.

Psychiatry has become a team effort and the social worker along with the nurse, the clinical psychologist, the occupational therapist and others, is an extremely valuable member of the team. Unfortunately her services are not always efficiently utilized. She should play an important part at all stages of the treatment process: for example, in obtaining background information regarding the illness and its possible precipitating factors in order to facilitate diagnosis; in providing support and practical help to the patient and the relatives; in preparing the patient for rehabilitation and in reducing environmental stresses which might adversely affect him when he returns home; and in supervising the patient and his family following his discharge from hospital. A good deal of social work, at whatever level, is concerned with the solving of problems: rather too often the social worker is given the most intractable problem when everyone else has tried and failed. When a case-load comes to consist of nothing but other people's "cast-outs", many of the social worker's special skills are wasted. We wish to stress the positive aspects of case-work and we believe that one of its main functions is to act as a counterbalance to the often too-clinical attitude we have already mentioned. The psychiatrist with an intelligent appreciation of the importance of social factors in mental illness will welcome the help given by his social worker colleagues.

Psychiatric Illness in the Community

There has always been an enormous amount of psychological disability in the community, some of it recognized as illness but much of it going without recognition. Most of these disturbances are psychoneurotic, and psychotic conditions form a relatively small proportion (though in absolute numbers they are very common). Before the neuroses came to be regarded as illnesses at all, most of these people got fairly short shrift from doctors and the general public alike and they often found it easier to suffer in silence, but nowadays people are much more ready to complain when they are psychologically unwell and, as well as this, expect to be made better. Most of these complaints are quite minor and relatively transient and in present circumstances general practitioners find themselves treating the great majority of such conditions. Usually only the most acute or the most persistent illnesses are referred to the psychiatrist, who therefore sees a highly selected group of patients.

In the general community a great variety of social workers and social agencies have the task of coping directly or indirectly with psychiatric illness and its effects. Unfortunately there is a tendency for all of us just to see our own little part of the overall problem of psychiatric illness and there is a great need for co-ordination of all these various services.

The psychiatrist of today spends a considerable part of his time working with outpatients. Many people can now be treated perfectly adequately without ever having to go into hospital: many others require only a comparatively short stay in hospital and then their treatment can be completed on an outpatient basis. The number of patients being treated psychiatrically continually rises but the total number of psychiatric hospital beds is falling as the need for prolonged institutional care diminishes. However, there is no doubt that the strenuous effort to keep patients in the community does produce social problems, often quite severe ones. The great majority of psychiatric patients do not cause social difficulties but there are those like the partially recovered schizophrenics who in previous times would have remained quietly locked away for the rest of their lives and who are now able to return home. Clinical recovery does not necessarily imply full recovery of social function and complicated provisions often have to be made for such people to remain in the community: even with such provisions the strain on the family and on the community may be severe.

It is not just psychiatry that is faced with this problem of social complications. Other medical specialists are coming to realize that physical illness cannot be regarded in isolation since inevitably it occurs in the setting of a human being; and the disease, the individual's emotions and his behaviour profoundly affect each other. The emotional element is often relatively unimportant (although there is evidence that it is easier to catch even a head-cold when one is depressed) but in some cases it is very important indeed and if it is neglected there is likely to be a most unsatisfactory response to treatment. As a simple example, it is known that some people who have had influenzal illness fail to "pick up" afterwards as they should. If the doctor does not recognize that these individuals may be depressed (because depression is quite a common sequel to influenza) they may go on being unwell long after recovery should have taken place and they remain "wide open" to a variety of illnesses for a considerable time. Recovery from an illness or an operation is delayed in some patients who are suffering from severe emotional problems: occasionally this is due to malingering, but most often it is a genuine delay brought about by psychological factors. It should be accepted that in these cases psychiatric treatment is almost as important as an antibiotic, a pain-killer or the surgeon's knife.

Too often the psychological element of a patient's physical complaint is only recognized late on when his illness has tended to become chronic. This should not happen: instead, the patient's mental state should be examined initially just as thoroughly as his physical state and any psychological disturbance treated promptly and efficiently. Not infrequently the cause of the trouble lies in some domestic or social problem and it is at this point that the social worker may become involved in the case. Her contribution may not only put a patient's mind at rest; it may materially shorten the duration of his illness and the length of his stay in hospital. But, to do this most efficiently, it is necessary for her to have a working knowledge of psychiatric principles in order to be able to cope with the situation and to communicate intelligently with her colleagues about this aspect of the patient's illness.

Psychiatric Knowledge for the Social Worker

A reasonable knowledge of psychiatry must be part of the equipment of anyone who is engaged in social work nowadays, but one reason why we set out to write this book was our concern that it should be *reasonable* knowledge. Psychiatry is a rapidly changing subject and its theoretical bases are continually altering. Concepts which were found satisfactory a few years ago can no longer explain many of the phenomena of mental illness that we now recognize. For example, some psychoanalytic theories have recently come under scrutiny and have been found wanting. Unfortunately many non-psychiatrists still cling to outmoded and inadequate theoretical beliefs, and as a result communication between the layman and the psychiatrist tends to break down. Sometimes the psychiatry which is taught to social workers is sectarian and out of date. We do not claim that this book is an authoritative account of up-to-the-minute psychiatry, but in it we try to present an eclectic view of psychiatry with no undue bias towards any particular school of psychiatric thought and which is realistically orientated towards modern practice.

There is a great need to bridge the gap which exists between the approach of the psychiatrist to mental illness and the approach of the social worker who may encounter mental illness in the course of case-work. As we have indicated, the psychiatrist's medical training orientates him towards the illness and his most fervent wish is to devise means by which a cure can be brought about as effectively as possible. Effectiveness need not imply impersonality, but sometimes things happen this way and the degree of impersonality in treatment may be increased by the large number of patients with whom the psychiatrist has to deal. In addition, the patient is usually seen in the artificial environment of the consulting room and it often takes an unusually hardy or indifferent patient to be himself in these circumstances.

These things are important but nothing is as important as the necessity for the patient to get better, and there is no question that modern treatments are proving more effective in dealing with most psychiatric illnesses. Nevertheless, since most of the recent developments in therapy have involved physical forms of treatment it is certainly important that the doctor should not forget the man who is ill in his keenness to treat the condition. Conversely the social worker should not ignore advances in the psychiatric field, especially where these advances are not of an exclusively psychological nature. Our services should be complementary and improvements in the one should be utilized to make the other more efficient.

The social worker does not need the doctor's clinical approach. Naturally her interest is in her client's recovery, but she does not have quite the same professional involvement as the psychiatrist in the need to cure the patient. She need not make such a definite distinction between health and disease: the doctor sees illness as a process which is foreign to the sufferer and which progressively encroaches on his well-being, whereas the social worker is more likely to see it in the dynamic terms of an individual's reaction to the environment and its stresses. By the nature of her work the social worker sees the patient not as a separate entity but as one unit in his family and wider social milieu: this attitude is commendable provided that she does not over-emphasize environment and under-estimate the importance of the sickness within the person.

The term patient is disliked by many people because of its connotations of sickness and treatment in bed. Nowadays, if a person has to be admitted to hospital we try to avoid treating him like a traditional patient. Very few psychiatric cases need bed treatment and we try to encourage the individual to retain his self-respect and his initiative because we know that loss of these can perpetuate and aggravate his illness. Our means for doing this are limited by the availability of staff and resources, but the principle of the therapeutic community in hospital has gained wide acceptance. But we must not forget that advances like this in our attitude to the mentally ill have only become possible with the increasing efficacy of psychiatric treatment.

Whether we call the person who needs our help a client or a patient is largely immaterial, but it is to his disadvantage if we cannot agree on ways to help him. It is no good pretending that differences of professional opinion do not arise between doctors and social workers, but when this happens the disagreement is often more apparent than real. It usually turns out that we are quarrelling over questions of definition or we are failing to appreciate that we are considering different aspects of the same illness situation. It is vital to the patient's interest that the social worker and the medical practitioner work in a team, if possible not duplicating each other's effort, but instead each providing a particular skill and concentrating on a particular aspect of the ill individual's problems. We have designed this book to provide factual information for social workers, but we hope that it will also demonstrate the need for psychiatrists and case-workers to communicate more readily and more efficiently for the ultimate benefit of the client-patient.

CHAPTER 2

Human Growth and Development

I. PHYSICAL DEVELOPMENT

When we come to study the development of the human being we are forced, for convenience' sake, to consider it as a series of processes, so that we talk of physical development, intellectual development, personality development and so on. It must be appreciated that this kind of division is largely artificial. The human individual grows and develops in a total way and all the component structures and functions of mind and body become inextricably interwoven as maturation occurs. The adult is the end-result of an extraordinarily complex developmental sequence and in the normal person there is an efficiency of function and of co-operation between different aspects of the organism which is utterly remarkable. As a result, an event which affects one part, directly or indirectly affects every other part. Activity of the mind invariably has some repercussion on the function of the body and vice versa. In order to have some understanding of the development of the personality we have to appreciate something of the body's development and some of its physiological characteristics. In this chapter we shall therefore present an extremely concise account of human physical development, concentrating on those aspects which are necessary as a background to the understanding of normal and abnormal personality development.

Normal Physical Development

The basic structural unit in the body is the CELL and it has been calculated that the average human body probably contains the astronomical number of some 60 million million cells. In a sense, each cell is a tiny living creature in its own right but in normal circumstances its functions are subservient to the organism as a whole and most cells have become so specialized that they can survive only by being part of the totality. Cells perform a variety of functions: some secrete hormones, some manufacture bone or hair; while some construct the bonding material which holds the components of the body together. The cells of the nervous system are specially constructed to transmit messages and those of the kidney are designed to eliminate waste products. In other bodily systems are cells which are concerned with reproduction, repelling invading microorganisms, ensuring adequate nutrition and so on. Most cells contain a nucleus and within the nucleus lie the CHROMOSOMES, of which there are normally 46 in each human cell. The chromosomes carry man's hereditary material, the genetic messages which are passed from generation to generation and which are necessary for the construction of a living and functioning being. Each separate message is carried on a GENE and a chromosome may be visualized as resembling a microscopic string of beads, each bead representing one gene. The chromosomes are arranged in 23 pairs and one of these pairs is responsible for determining the sex of the individual. In a female the two sex chromosomes are identical in appearance and each is known as an X-chromosome. In the male there is one X-chromosome and a smaller Y-chromosome.

When cells divide, every chromosome splits into two so that the resulting pair of "daughter" cells each has its full complement of genetic material. Most of the cells in a given individual will therefore have the same genetic constitution but the germ cells are strikingly different. These are the cells which are involved in the process of reproduction and in their formation a complicated process of redistribution of genetic material occurs, with the eventual result that each germ cell contains only 23 chromosomes—22 somatic chromosomes plus one sex chromosome. In females the sex chromosomes can only be of the X type because the female possesses no Y. In males the germ cell may contain either an X or a Y. It is thus the male who determines the sex of the child and this determination occurs at the moment of conception.

Fertilization of the Ovum

The male germ cell, the sperm, is a minute, tadpole-shaped body which is capable of free and vigorous movement. The female germ cell, or ovum, is very much larger and is not mobile of its own accord. When coitus has taken place, enormous numbers of sperm are liberated into the female genital tract and they pass actively up through the uterus. Each month an ovum is released from the ovary and is transferred towards the uterus in preparation for fertilization. Encounter between sperm and ovum usually occurs in the Fallopian tube which connects ovary and uterus and it is usually the fittest and most vigorous sperm which is successful in bringing about fertilization. It penetrates the outer membrane of the ovum and thereafter the nuclei of the two germ cells fuse, forming a single cell which has its full complement of 46 chromosomes. The genetic sex will depend on whether the union has produced an XX or an XY constitution. The fertilized ovum then begins to undergo repeated cell-division as it passes down into the cavity of the uterus, eventually to become implanted in the internal surface of the wall of that organ.

Fertilization is not possible all the time in the human female. Every four weeks or so during her reproductive life the woman undergoes a series of physical changes controlled by sex hormones which are secreted within her body. These changes constitute the menstrual cycle and each cycle represents a preparation of the uterus for the anticipated reception of a fertilized ovum. If fertilization does not occur, the lining of the uterus is cast off and disposed of in the menstrual flow and the process then recommences. Approximately half-way between successive menses an ovum is released from one or other ovary and then the woman is fertile until the next menstrual period occurs. (Along with the physical changes which occur, as a result of hormonal influences there may also be quite marked mood changes during the cycle, with an especial tendency towards anxiety and depression in the pre-menstrual phase.)

The female is born with her full complement of ova already

present in the ovaries and during her reproductive years perhaps 400 of these are released. In the male the situation is quite different. Sperm are manufactured continuously in prodigious quantities and a single emission may contain almost 500 million of them. A normal man is physically capable of reproducing at any time. He has no equivalent of the menstrual cycle or the female menopause.

Development of the Embryo

After it becomes embedded in the uterine lining the fertilized ovum continues its rapid and complex process of cell-division. It soon converts itself into a solid sphere and then into a hollow cyst. After this, one part of the cyst-wall begins to form the embryo proper and the rest develops into the various structures that will protect and nourish the embryo during the ensuing 40 weeks of development in the uterus. These structures include the membranes which surround the embryo, and the placenta, the organ which is responsible for the exchange of oxygen and nutrition from mother to child and of waste products in the opposite direction.

During these following 9 months the embryo develops from a tiny mass of cells to an eminently recognizable human being. It has often been pointed out that during the early part of embryonic development a rapid recapitulation of the evolutionary process occurs. At first the embryo resembles a flat-worm, then it becomes more like a round-worm. Soon after that it becomes fish-like, with gills and a tail, and then the gills close over and the tail is absorbed just like a frog. Thereafter the mammalian form and ultimately the human form become evident. During the intra-uterine period the embryo receives all its nutrition and oxygen from the mother via the placenta. It floats in a shock-proof fluid environment and the mother's body provides protection until the infant has become mature enough to leave the womb. Sometimes, for one reason or another, the pregnancy is a failure. In some cases this is due to an inherent fault in the embryo, in others it is due to inadequacy of the uterine lining to sustain the pregnancy or to damage caused to the embryo when the placenta has been unable to prevent the passage of a harmful substance from the mother's blood-stream. Whatever the cause, the frequent result is a spontaneous abortion, and in this country at least one pregnancy in ten ends this way.

The Foetus

After 8 weeks the embryo is still tiny but is a recognizable human being with most of the adult body structures present in primitive form. From now on the embryo is known as the foetus and until birth occurs at or around the 40th week of gestation it grows enormously in size and there is increasing complexity of body structure and the development of a variety of body functions. The nervous system shares in this rapid process so that at birth the brain has its full life-time complement of nerve cells, there is a well-developed peripheral nervous system to enable the brain to control movement and to register sensory impressions, and there is an autonomic nervous system by which the brain can supervise the body's internal activities.

Before the pregnancy is half-way through, the foetus begins to show movement and the mother becomes aware of the unborn child's "quickening". Psychologists have performed experiments which show that the foetus is capable of responding to external stimuli by making movements, but as well as this it is able to move spontaneously. Its heart beats regularly and before birth takes place most of the vital functions are well established so that the infant has a chance of survival even if it is born prematurely. The premature infant is very unlikely to survive if it has not reached the 28th week of gestation, but its chances of living and developing normally increase rapidly the nearer to term it is.

Normally birth does not occur until the foetus is mature enough to stand the rigours of the birth process and life thereafter. When this stage of development has been reached, the mother goes into labour and the infant is delivered. As the birth canal is relatively narrow the head of the infant has to adapt its shape slightly in order to pass through. This usually causes no damage but occasionally may result in brain injury in the infant. Brain damage may also occur if the labour is prolonged and the child is temporarily starved of oxygen. However, the vast majority of babies survive delivery without harm and immediately after birth they begin to breathe. The umbilical cord connecting the child to the placenta, and through which nourishment and oxygen have passed, is severed. A number of physical changes rapidly take place within the child to enable it to adapt to its new-found independence. Once the delivery is complete, the placenta separates from the wall of the uterus and is expelled as the afterbirth.

Development following Birth

When it is born a normal child weighs between 7 lb and 8 lb, but there is a wide range of normality. This weight will be doubled by the end of the first 6 months and trebled by the end of the first year. The length of the newborn infant is about 20 inches and this takes about 4 years to double itself. At birth the baby can see but cannot hear, and taste and smell are not developed until 2 or 3 days later. There is a very limited range of activities which includes the ability to suck, to draw attention to itself by crying, and to excrete. There are also certain reflex activities such as grasping and making walking movements which serve little real purpose in the human infant and probably represent an evolutionary survival.

The first year of life is a period of rapid physical development during which the baby's muscles become stronger and his movements more skilled. He learns to hold up his head, then sit up (at first with support and then by himself), crawl and finally stand with support. These motor skills develop in a fairly definite order and within a reasonably fixed period of time. While recognizing that there is a range of normality, it is still possible to gauge a child's rate of development by noting the ages at which he passes these various "milestones". At first, nutrition is obtained entirely from milk and in primitive societies breast-feeding may go on for a year or more. At the present time in our own society mixed feeding is usually introduced by the 3rd or 4th month and weaning is likely to be completed by the 7th or 8th month.

As the infant is growing in length and weight he is also maturing physically. At the time of birth certain organs contain as many cells as they will ever have: we have mentioned the brain in this respect and it is also true of the heart. In many other tissues, cell division continues and may go on throughout life, so that, for example, bone, connective tissue and skin are capable of expanding as the child develops. Somewhere between the age of 5 months and 9 months the teeth begin to appear and these milk teeth continue to erupt until about the middle of the 3rd year. The presence of teeth naturally enables the infant to tackle a much more varied diet. In order to ensure adequate growth food has to be plentiful and must include essential proteins, fats and carbohydrate as well as minerals and vitamins.

Soon after his first birthday, the baby should begin to take a few steps on his own and after this he gradually becomes an active toddler. From this time till the onset of puberty there is continuing growth and an increase in power, skill and co-ordination. There are slight developmental differences between the sexes and girls tend to be taller before adolescence. Then, as puberty is reached there is a spectacular spurt in growth and physical development.

Puberty and Adolescence

The age at which puberty appears varies with the individual. Girls usually reach this stage before boys but there is again a wide range of normality for both sexes. Normally the girl begins to mature sexually between the 10th and 11th years and the boy a year or two later. In the two sexes the really intense period of growth lasts about 2 years and during this time the boys overtake the girls in height. The onset of physical maturation is accompanied in the girl by the menarche (the appearance of menstruation), but there is no such definite incident to mark it in the boy's case. The fact that menstruation is occurring does not mean that the girl is immediately fertile because for the first year or two she does not ovulate: in other words, no eggs are released from the ovaries during this time. It is well known that the age of the menarche is steadily decreasing in

Western countries and this appears to be related to improving standards of health and nutrition.

The physical changes which occur at puberty and during adolescence are spectacular. The height rapidly increases, the childish appearance is lost and a much more adult physique appears. In boys, the muscles develop greatly, the shoulders widen and the bones become more solid. At first there is a tendency for growth to outstrip energy and skill and this accounts for the adolescent's proverbial clumsiness and his rapidly alternating phases of furious energy and listlessness. The voice deepens as the larynx becomes larger. The gonads or sex glands (in males, the testes) enlarge and begin to produce sperm and also increased amounts of male sex hormone. There is rapid development of the secondary sexual characteristics, with enlargement of the penis and growth of facial and axillary hair. At this time the boy will begin to have penile erections (which at first he may find alarming and embarrassing) and he may also have seminal emissions which to begin with usually occur involuntarily during sleep.

The girl also displays rapid physical development. Her sex glands, the ovaries, secrete large quantities of female sex hormones under whose influence her body assumes the typical feminine contours, largely due to the deposition of subcutaneous fat. The breasts and nipples enlarge, the genital tract matures and the pubic and axillary hair appears. In both sexes all of these changes are largely under the control of the pituitary gland, an organ about the size of a pea which is situated below the base of the brain and which is itself controlled to some extent by certain areas of the brain. At puberty the pituitary begins to secrete a number of hormones, these being chemical substances which pass into the blood-stream and are carried to other organs where they have some specific effect. These hormones are responsible for growth, for the appropriate secondary sexual development of male and female and for fertility. Eventually, by their effects on the bones, the pituitary hormones and the sex hormones will determine the cessation of growth, which usually occurs in late adolescence or young adulthood.

Adult Life

After puberty and during adolescence there is a process of physical maturation and consolidation. The individual becomes a fully functional adult who is capable of reproduction. In many ways he has reached his physical peak by his early twenties, at which time his reactions are quickest and his motor skills and co-ordination are at their height. Thereafter there is a slow but steady decline in physical performance, though this is compensated for for a considerable time by increasing experience and greater powers of endurance (which is partly a psychological effect). Many of the tissues of the body become gradually less resilient and less capable of effecting repair, a process most obviously noticeable in the skin, which slowly loses its suppleness and elasticity. By the middle forties, the individual is usually leading a much more sedentary life than in youth and as a result he tends to put on some extra weight.

At about this time the woman goes through the menopause, the phase which marks the end of her reproductive life. This is once more under the control of the pituitary, which ceases to produce certain hormones, and the result is the cessation of ovulation and of menstruation. The latter sometimes disappears quite suddenly or it may become scantier and scantier till, after a time, it stops. Due to the chemical changes which occur within the woman's body at this time she may experience certain physical symptoms such as flushing, perspiring and malaise and the mood may be somewhat unstable till the menopause is complete. Despite this and the numerous old wives' tales about the "change of life", the majority of women pass through the stage without excessive physical or psychological disturbance. As we have already indicated, the male has no such well-marked end to his reproductive era.

With further progression into middle age there is more of the gradual physical deterioration which involves every part of the body though not necessarily all at the same rate. Each individual has his own rate of aging and individual organs also have their own speeds at which they degenerate. The body's metabolism becomes rather slower and the tendency to put on weight continues as activity decreases. The arteries become less flexible and less capable of carrying adequate blood supplies to the tissues, which are relatively starved of oxygen and nutrient substances. The tissues in turn may atrophy and this sometimes happens very strikingly in the brain, with resultant mental deterioration. On the whole, however, the process is a fairly slow and imperceptible one and since it is universal it must be regarded as a physiological, rather than a pathological, condition.

Old Age

The person gradually passes into old age, when the all-round effects of physical deterioration become very much more noticeable. Chronological age has little meaning by this time because some people are senile before they are sixty while others are fresh and vigorous in their seventies. In general, however, the old person is unmistakably weaker and slower, his brain has aged and mental functions like memory and learning are impaired. His bones are more brittle and resistance to physical disease becomes reduced. Eventually, death occurs, either as part of the process of failing function or due to some disease which has attacked the weakened body. The biblical life-span of three-score years and ten is still a fairly reasonable one to expect, and indeed nowadays many more people can assume that they will reach it because of the greatly reduced mortality rates among infants and young people in civilized countries.

The Interplay of Heredity and Environment in Normal Physical Development

The individual's genetic constitution determines that he will be a human being with all the physical attributes that this implies. So far as may be determined the ultimate basis of all events within a human being, whether somatic or psychological, is at a physical level and the fact that these events can occur is ultimately dependent on genetic factors. The genetic plan is laid down at conception but this does not mean that its results cannot be modified. The plan should rather be regarded as a potential which may or may not be realized according to a variety of effects, many of them environmental, and these effects begin to modify the organism's development right from the beginning. For example, within the uterus the amount of available nutrition will play a great part in determining the rate at which weight-gain progresses. If nutrition is poor, foetal development may be permanently affected, and if it is very poor, abortion may well occur. Sometimes, the foetus may be affected by certain diseases, or chemical substances which pass through the placenta and cause harm. Rubella (German Measles) and Thalidomide are well-known examples of this type of event. Whatever the cause, if the developing brain is affected the child's intellect and personality may be permanently impaired. Prematurity and its complications tend to have an adverse effect on both physical and psychological development.

After birth there is a long and complex interaction between heredity and environment. Adequate nutrition and good general conditions will ensure maximal growth rates, an early onset of puberty, greater strength and stature and, on the whole, higher intelligence. As a rule, one's genetic constitution sets a limit which can be reached but cannot be passed and this limit varies for different people. Under more or less identical conditions of development, different individuals will show marked inequalities of height, weight, motor skills and aptitudes, intelligence and capability. Even the duration of the life-span is to a considerable degree determined by heredity and there are almost certainly important genetic factors present in some of the psychiatric illnesses. We have no wish to deny the importance of environmental factors which play an enormous part in human development but we would emphasize that in assessing a person's physical or mental state, the social worker should give hereditary and constitutional factors their due place.

The Sexual Function

Since two sexes obviously exist we tend to take this fact for granted and not question the need for there being males and females. Nor do we usually bother to enquire why sexual union is required before a new individual is conceived. Many humble creatures reproduce satisfactorily simply by dividing themselves in two, so why do higher animals almost invariably reproduce by sexual means?

There are two main reasons and the first is obvious. An extremely simple organism can divide itself with comparatively little difficulty but a more complex organism would experience very great mechanical difficulty in achieving this. Secondly, and much more importantly, sexual reproduction allows for very much greater variability in the characteristics of the offspring since the latter is the result of inheritance from two sources rather than one. This provides a great evolutionary advantage. Evolution has been a continual struggle by life-forms for increasing mastery over the environment. Simple organisms can be biologically highly successful but their range of operations is usually very limited. Genetically, their offspring are just "chips off the old block" and this type of reproduction gives little scope for the development of versatility or the ability to cope with changing environmental conditions. Occasionally a genetic mutation occurs and the offspring then differs in some significant respect from its "parent", but most mutations are harmful and it is only a tiny proportion which confer benefit on the species, so this form of evolution is extremely slow and inflexible.

Creatures with a sexual form of reproduction can also experience gene mutation, but it is obvious that if two individuals share their genetic material during the process of conception, then the possibility of variability and adaptability of the species is much increased. In the process of formation of the germ cells there is a complicated "shuffling" of the genetic material and this means that no two people can ever be genetically identical unless they result from the splitting of a fertilized ovum, as happens with identical twins. Not all genetic combinations will be advantageous, but with the infinite number of variations possible there are bound to be some which give the offspring an extra chance of success.

Mating

In order that the germ cells of the two sexes may unite, mating must take place and this must be a desirable activity or else the species would soon become extinct. In the human female, coitus can be comparatively passive, but in the male it is an active physical process. The woman may indulge in sexual activity before she has reached the age of being fertile, during the infertile portion of her menstrual cycle between menstruation and ovulation, and when she has become infertile after the menopause, so fertility is not a prerequisite for coitus. This is true for the male also, but since his role is essentially an active one there are several limiting factors to his mating capabilities. For him, sexual intercourse is usually possible only after puberty when the penis has enlarged sufficiently to enable penetration to occur. He must be sexually aroused and only then will erection of the penis occur and coitus be able to take place. If, however, he is impotent so that he cannot obtain an erection in the sexual situation, sexual intercourse is virtually impossible.

After penetration, the male achieves orgasm which coincides with the seminal emission. The semen contains the sperm which are thus liberated into the vagina and which then begin to move actively up through the uterus on their journey to fertilize the ovum. The female orgasm is more a psychological than a physical reaction, though none the less real for that. Ideally the man and woman should experience orgasm more or less simultaneously. Afterwards there is a variable period during which the male is unable to have further intercourse, but the female is capable of multiple orgasms if sufficiently stimulated.

The purpose of coitus is, of course, conception, but in human beings it is also employed as a powerful source of physical and psychological pleasure, though it can equally be a source of severe frustration. Its effectiveness as a means of reproduction can be interrupted by a variety of factors. Infertility in either partner is one such factor. There are numerous forms of sexual disorder which prevent normal sexual relations from taking place and most of these are psychological—for example, frigidity and impotence (see Chapter 6)—though some are of a physical nature. It is noticeable that our species protects itself, since the most seriously damaged individuals in human society (for example, the low-grade mentally subnormal, the severely physically handicapped, the schizophrenic) are often impotent or infertile. Nowadays we are deliberately interfering with conception, though not with coitus, by means of contraception. One side-effect of this is that many more women can now begin to enjoy sexual relations more fully, because they are no longer haunted by the fear of repeated pregnancies.

A great many legends exist regarding women and sex. For instance, it is not so very long since it was believed in our society that women neither could nor should enjoy sexual relations. The female was expected to be a passive sexual partner and this often resulted in complete failure of satisfaction for her. Nowadays we know that women are equally capable of sexual passion, but it is also realized that the two sexes are sexually aroused in rather different ways and sometimes by different circumstances. Men are usually more rapidly aroused by the presence or even the thought of a desired female. Women are rather more slowly aroused and their sexual emotion tends much more to be part of a total emotional situation, but once they have become sexually excited their feelings are just as powerful as the man's. Unfortunately, many men equate satisfaction in coitus with the achievement of their own orgasm and through insensitivity or clumsiness they may prevent their partners from achieving equal satisfaction. A great many women who are not truly frigid have never really experienced orgasm for this reason and many have become repelled by sexual intercourse because of repeated frustrations. Now that sexual matters are much more freely discussed and sex has become a sufficiently respectable subject for research there is a much greater opportunity to elicit the causes of sexual disorders and to treat them on a rational basis.

Physical Maldevelopment

This is a huge subject and we can only touch upon it in this volume. We have already mentioned that physical growth and development can be halted or diverted at any stage by a multiplicity of influences. Within the uterus the foetus may be adversely affected by genetic defects, lack of nutrition, lack of oxygen or damage by infections or chemical substances. As a result the child may be born damaged or incomplete in some way, perhaps mentally defective, crippled due to some deformity or lacking a vital organ. After birth, possibly harmful influences are plentiful. Adverse genetic influences may continue to make their presence known through life and malnutrition may cause stunting and physical disease. Injury and illness can cause damage to individual parts of the body or to the entire individual. Intrinsic failures of development may occur as, for example, when the pituitary fails to secrete its hormones and dwarfism results.

The earlier in the process of development the damage is done the more general is the resulting disorder likely to be. Each stage and age has its own typical patterns of disease and injury and the two sexes have their own peculiar morbidity patterns, but whenever development is interfered with, the individual's whole being is affected. It is never enough to consider only the physical aspects of maldevelopment or disease. The patient has to attempt to compensate psychologically for his handicap and he may or may not be successful in doing this. In some cases, he may even over-compensate to some degree and become one of those people who develop a striking talent in defiance of the disability. If he is less fortunate he may simply develop an obsessive feeling of unhappiness with his lot. It is, therefore, always necessary when making a physical or psychological assessment of a person to take into account any notable handicaps and to discover how well or otherwise he has learned to cope with these.

CHAPTER 3

Human Growth and Development

II. PERSONALITY DEVELOPMENT

It is virtually impossible to define what we mean by "personality". The word is derived from the Latin *persona*, which was the mask traditionally worn by an actor in classical times to represent a character in a play. From this limited usage it came to mean the "face" that the individual presents to the world at large. We shall use the word personality in an even wider sense, to include all the psychological and social attributes which go to make up the individual being. The personality is a dynamic structure, constantly interacting with the environment and constantly being modified by circumstances. In order to understand a man's personality we have to have a knowledge of his developmental background and of the ways in which he and his environment influence each other.

In the previous chapter we talked about the effects of evolution and of heredity and we considered the process of human physical development from conception onwards. Even before birth the foetus is subjected to numerous extraneous influences, but of course it has only a very limited capacity for reacting to them. After birth, the opportunities to interact with the surroundings are greatly enhanced and obviously the surroundings themselves and the events which occur within them are much richer in variety than anything which can take place within the womb. The new-born child has a very limited range of actual capabilities, but its potential for development is enormous. This potential will be realized to a greater or lesser extent as a result of the child's inborn drives and the effects of the great variety of outside influences which these encounter. As a consequence of this developmental process each individual comes to have a unique personality and there are many theories which try to explain exactly how this happens.

Some Theories of Personality

During the nineteenth century there was considerable dispute between those who believed that personality was an indivisible entity which could only be understood as a whole and those others (mainly psychologists) who claimed that it was possible to analyse personality into its constituent parts. The former group took the somewhat mystical approach that the personality was greater than the sum of its parts and so the study of these parts was relatively meaningless because they could never completely explain the whole. The others insisted that there was nothing inherently mysterious about the personality, though it was admittedly highly complex. Gradually this latter opinion gained ground and when Darwin's theories of evolution appeared they greatly aided this view. Many people became convinced that survival of the species was the most important driving force in living beings, and survival of the individual was regarded mainly as a factor which subserved this purpose. Psychological processes might promote survival, provided they were efficient and well integrated in the individual's total nature. It became apparent that man's psychological constitution was unique only in that it was better developed than that of lower creatures and this dispelled much of the semi-mystical aura which had always surrounded the workings of the mind. Borrowing a concept from contemporary physics, nineteenth-century psychologists visualized the organism as a type of energy system which required fuel in the form of food and was able to discharge energy in the shape of physical, emotional and intellectual activity. They pointed out that we could only dispel as much energy as we had received, though obviously we could alter the form it took—for example, changing physical to intellectual energy.

Medical psychology of that time was greatly in need of a theory to explain the phenomenon of mental illness. It had usually been assumed till then that it was either a mysterious visitation upon the individual or else evidence of some form of hereditary degeneration. Freud's theories seemed not only to explain how personality developed but also how psychiatric disorders appeared as a pathological outgrowth of this developmental process. In addition, they bestowed respectability upon psychoneurotic disorders because he showed that it was possible to regard these as illnesses with a cause and a pattern of development, whereas previously they had been condemned as manifestations of moral weakness. Freud stressed the importance of adverse early life experiences in the genesis of many psychiatric conditions and his views still influence our ideas regarding the development and maldevelopment of the personality. However, as we shall mention, many of his assertions have had to be modified with the passage of time. Freud was a physician and his clients were almost invariably people with psychiatric disturbances. To construct a theory of normal personality growth he had to rely on his observations of the abnormal, and infer from these the patterns of normality. Since his patients were always adults, his information on childhood events was entirely retrospective and he himself came to appreciate how fallacious such information could sometimes be. It is indeed paradoxical that so many of our views on psychological normality have been derived from studies of the abnormal, but fortunately the modern trend is towards the direct observation of children to ascertain the actual events and sequences which occur in the process of personality maturation.

Psychoanalytic theory assumes that, at birth, the infant possesses a small number of instinctual drives which are determined mainly by hereditary factors. These instincts appear to have an innate tendency to develop and diversify and, as Freud originally conceived of the process, this occurred in a rather predestined and mechanical way, though environmental influences were acknowledged to play a considerable modifying role. The basic instinct was the one considered most necessary for preservation of the species, the sexual instinct, and all the others were regarded as derivations from this. Since this idea was propounded in Victorian times when there was an extremely puritanical public attitude towards sexual matters, it is hardly surprising that psychoanalysis met with such furious opposition at first. When Freud pursued his hypotheses further he caused even greater dismay because, in his theory of infantile sexuality, he pointed out that children were not the angelic creatures of traditional nineteenth-century belief. Instead, they were endowed with sexual feelings from earliest infancy. This view can now be widely accepted, but then it appeared revolting to many people.

The concept of the unconscious mind had been current before Freud's time, but he drew attention to its great importance in mental functioning. Despite much evidence to the contrary it had usually been argued that man was a rational being whose conscious self was largely in control of his "baser" unconscious self. Psychoanalysis pointed out that, in fact, the unconscious occupied a very large part of the mind and that consciousness was a small, if highly important, part of the total mental apparatus. Freud also suggested that the mind could be regarded as operating in three main compartments which he named the *Id*, the *Ego* and the *Superego*. (When using these terms it is as well to remember that they do not relate to underlying anatomical structures within the brain. Rather, they form a convenient schema by the use of which we may find the mind's workings more intelligible.) The id, ego and superego are not static structures. There is a dynamic relationship between them so that an event in one is bound to have repercussions in the others. There is also a developmental relationship. The id is the undifferentiated, instinctual aspect of mental function which is found in the very young infant: it represents the predominance of emotion over intellect. The ego develops after birth; it draws much of its energy from the id and it gradually comes to control the more primitive instinctual functions. The superego develops even later and is largely an off-shoot of the ego. It acts as a conscience and to some extent it is responsible for the individual's social behaviour.

As the personality matures, the instincts are brought ever more under the bidding of the ego but they are never destroyed. They remain, mostly at an unconscious level, in order to provide much of the individual's drive and mental energy. The id operates on the

Pleasure Principle. In other words, it does not recognize the need to postpone gratification and any psychic discomfort must be immediately relieved by some form of pleasure-giving or tension-relieving activity. The ego, on the other hand, works on the *Reality Principle* and is prepared to delay the gratification of instinctual impulses in order to achieve some end. Much of the activity of the ego also goes on at an unconscious level but generally its material is more accessible to consciousness than that of the id. Within the ego-structure there are a number of defence mechanisms which, operating unconsciously, enable the individual to adapt to reality and which filter the impact of instinctual demands on the one hand and the impact of the external environment on the other. By this means the person is able to maintain his mental equilibrium in ever-changing circumstances. In traditional psychoanalysis the ideal mental state was thought to be a Nirvana-like tranquillity and the human mind was visualized as constantly striving to combat tension and anxiety. Nowadays this view is not widely accepted as there is evidence that man possesses a built-in quota of restlessness and exploratory activity which is necessary for his mental well-being.

The ego–defences are a series of unconscious mechanisms which, as we have just mentioned, filter reality, but are also capable of denying or falsifying it. *Denial* is an extremely important defence and when something is too unpleasant to be borne the mind is able to pretend that the difficulty does not exist. Other ways of denying the unacceptable include *Repression*, when the mind pushes something out of consciousness so that it is "forgotten" (it is actually still present in the unconscious); and *Suppression*, when the same process is carried out at a conscious level. When a severe emotional conflict arises at some stage of development and is not fully resolved, the unresolved feelings are said to have become *Fixated* at that particular level of development. In later life, if the individual is under stress and mature methods of coping with this have been unsuccessful, he may, temporarily, return to a less mature form of emotional behaviour, a defence which is known as *Regression*. From practical experience we know that regression can be a very effective method of problem-solving. For example, an individual being assailed by another may find resistance unavailing and may then begin to weep, which is a very childish way to behave. Nevertheless, the helplessness and the tears often arouse pity in the other person and thus the situation may be resolved. There are various other ego-defences, but we shall mention just one more, that of *Projection*. This is a fairly primitive form of thinking in which the individual believes that his own thoughts and feelings are present in the mind of another and it is akin to the thinking of the child who thinks that people are good or bad according to the way in which he perceives them. In the adult, an unacceptable thought or feeling is easier to accept if the responsibility for it is placed on someone else. As an example, a man may entertain sexual fantasies towards some unattainable woman and these feelings may be against his moral code. It is much easier to accept the situation if he projects his feelings on to her and comes to believe that she is trying to seduce him. Then he can deny his own emotions and also indulge in the luxury of condemning someone else's moral laxity.

All of these ego defence mechanisms constitute part of normal mental activity and without them life would be harsh and unbearable. However, reality can be denied too much and when the ego-defences are over-employed the individual may lose his grip on circumstances and the result, as we shall show in a subsequent chapter, may be the development of a psychiatric illness.

Instincts continually attempt to manifest themselves in behaviour and it is largely by patterns of behaviour that we judge an individual's personality. In psychoanalysis the primitive and undifferentiated sexual instinct is equated with the life-force, and development of the personality is seen as an evolutionary process with procreation as its ultimate aim. (In order to explain the phenomenon of suicide, Freud postulated a corresponding death-instinct but this hypothesis was not widely accepted, even by psychoanalysts.) The first few years of life are vital in establishing personality features and in determining whether the individual will become a stable and well-functioning adult or not. The early development of the emotions falls into stages which Freud designated according to the region of the body which provides the greatest degree of pleasurable sensation at that particular time. Since the very young infant receives most of his gratification by way of his mouth he is said to be in the *Oral Phase*. Later, feeding activity becomes less predominant and the child develops greater awareness of its excretory processes. During this *Anal Phase*, pleasure (which is regarded as the forerunner of sexual pleasure) is largely derived from sensations arising in the lower bowel. Thereafter the *Phallic Phase* is reached and the genital organs become the prime source of erotic pleasure. Around the age of 4 years or so the child enters the *Oedipal Stage*, and if emotional maturation is not hindered at this point, the *Genital Phase* of sexual development is attained. Now there is emphasis on the psychological as well as on the physical aspects of sexuality and the basis for normal adult sexual behaviour has been laid down. If emotional development is held up at any one of these phases, this may determine to a considerable extent the individual's subsequent personality structure and also the pattern of his sexuality. If emotion is fixated completely at an immature level he may utterly fail to develop adult personality features, but if fixation is only partial, a superficial degree of maturity may be possible. However, under conditions of stress there will always be a tendency to regress to the emotional level at which fixation has occurred.

As the sexual instinct is maturing, all the other facets of personality are also developing. The child requires constant contact with other human beings with whom he may *Identify*. At first, most of his contact is with mother, then this extends to father, other members of the immediate family, then to relatives, friends and acquaintances. All the time he is modelling himself on them. Alongside this process he is also learning unconsciously to *Displace* his instinctual drives. This means that he uses his various defence mechanisms to temper the crudity of his instincts and to make the process of maturation easier and less distressing.

A great deal of Freudian psychological theory has become part of current thinking and many of its concepts retain their validity. It should be recognized that it is essentially a system of medical psychology, devised to explain mental illness, but its formulations have not always proved adequate in the field of normal human psychology. It is frequently criticized because it consists largely of explanations with very little experimental evidence to back these up. Nowadays there is a much greater tendency to rely on the tests of observation and experiment and psychoanalytic concepts are being subjected to closer scrutiny than ever before. They cannot fail to be the better for this. Meantime, there have been numerous developments and offshoots from Freud's original hypotheses and in recent years orthodox psychoanalysis has laid a great deal more emphasis on the importance of ego-function than he himself did.

Psychoanalysis has provided the starting point for a number of significant contributions to knowledge concerning personality development. We can discuss only a very few of these contributions in the space available to us and since this book is concerned with psychiatry we have deliberately chosen to mention the work of individuals who were primarily involved in the therapeutic aspects of the subject.

C. G. Jung (1875–1961) was originally a follower of Freud but came to disagree with him on a number of fundamental issues, one being the belief that psychoanalysis placed too much emphasis on the importance of the sexual instinct. From the point of view of treatment, Jung's contributions have not been especially valuable, though a number of psychiatrists still practise *Analytical Psychology,* the Jungian form of interpretative therapy. However, some of his concepts have entered current use and it is to him that we owe the term "Complex" as applied to a phrase like "Inferiority Complex". This does not have a very precise meaning, but it implies a constellation of emotions, thoughts, perceptions and memories which have some common focus or theme and which exist in that part of the unconscious closest to consciousness. Jung also introduced the concept that personalities fall into two general groups. On one side are the people who are predominantly *Extraverted* and whose prevailing attitudes are those of external action and sociability, and on the other those who are *Introverted* and who show marked traits of introspection and self-sufficiency. This idea of personality types has led to many useful attempts to classify personality accurately, but on the whole Jung's concepts tend to shade into metaphysics or mysticism. They may have some value to other disciplines but they have not proved generally helpful in psychiatric treatment.

Alfred Adler (1870–1937) was another colleague who broke away from Freud to found his own school, that of *Individual Psychology*. Adler took an important theoretical step forward when he pointed out that it was not possible to understand human personality development unless one viewed it within a social context. Man is an inherently social being and much of his behaviour is determined by his contact with other people. Like Jung, Adler placed less stress on the sexual drive than did Freud, and instead he contended that aggression was the basic instinct. By aggression he did not simply mean hostile behaviour, but rather a striving for superiority or self-completion. According to him, the human being always starts from a position of inferiority as an infant and aggression is the force which enables him to rise above this level. Because of social pressures the aggression is prevented from being simply naked self-interest and instead it is sublimated or subjugated, often in a way that proves useful to society. Another of Adler's concepts was that of *Organ Inferiority*. He suggested that most people were born with some degree of insufficiency of body or mind and that in the course of development of the physique or the personality a process of "compensation" takes place whereby the healthy aspects of the individual make up for the deficiency, whatever it happens to be. Thus a man with crippled legs might develop especially strong arms to aid his mobility or he might strive to succeed in the intellectual sphere to make up for his physical disability. Although on the whole Adler's work has not had a great deal of influence on psychiatric treatment his theory of organ inferiority was a forerunner of the psychosomatic concept, because it implied that a physical disability could demand psychological compensation and vice versa. In addition, the emphasis he placed on man's social instincts made him a pioneer of social psychiatry.

Harry Stack Sullivan (1892–1949) is notable mainly for his *Interpersonal Theory*, which went even further than Adler's views on social functioning. Sullivan declared that personality cannot be understood at all unless in the context of the interpersonal situation. An individual's personality exists only as it relates to other people and its development is regarded mostly as a result of social influences which may be beneficial or adverse. In any situation where two people come in contact each is bound to affect the other, and Sullivan emphasized that in the treatment situation both patient and therapist react on each other, so that the latter cannot be the mere onlooker and interpreter that psychoanalysis originally visualized. This particular assertion is now widely accepted but Sullivan's theories are in general somewhat extreme. They are shared to a considerable extent by the school of existential psychology, which insists that a man can only be understood as he stands in relation to time and his environment. Certainly it can be shown experimentally that if an individual is completely cut off from company and from all forms of sensory stimulus there is usually a severe degree of ego-disruption after a time. This usually only occurs in extreme and highly artificial circumstances and we believe that there is a certain structure to the normal personality which makes it unique and recognizable in most situations.

In recent years there has tended to be a synthesis of views on personality growth. Useful concepts have been adopted from various sources and have been put to the experimental test. The trend is away from a rigid, doctrinaire approach and also away from the rather mechanistic theories of personality development which prevailed for so many years. A great deal of useful and verifiable material is being contributed by subjects like psychology, biology and ethology. Within the psychoanalytic movement there has been a considerable divergence of interests, some mainly theoretical (for example, the Kleinian School) and others more experimental and more prepared to co-operate with disciplines outside psychiatry. Nowadays it has come to be realized that findings must never be distorted to fit a preconceived theoretical framework but must be allowed to speak for themselves.

It is fairly obvious that children vary widely in their capabilities and their activities from the moment of birth. Freud considered that their activities were directed mainly towards the ultimate achievement of procreation and, at the level of the individual, the attainment of emotional equilibrium. The environment appeared to be almost an accidental intrusion into this scheme of things. Now we have to accept that mind, body and environment all have their important part to play in the development of the personality.

Further Development of the Personality

We have already given some account of the child's earliest development. At the age of four or thereabouts the little boy undergoes a process of emotional change during the Oedipal stage and this results in his largely discarding his infantile sexual yearnings towards his mother. If all has gone well he is able to identify with his father and thus the basis is formed for his adult sexual role. The little girl goes through a similar process (sometimes known as the *Electra stage*) in order to become fully identified with her female role. Thereafter, until the onset of puberty the child undergoes a phase during which there is rapid intellectual development and emotional maturation but, in Western society at least, relatively little overt sexual activity. Because of the comparative absence of sexuality this phase is known as the *Latency Period*. During it the child becomes progressively more able to think in abstract terms and the superego begins to assume its adult form so that moral judgement is no longer a simple dependence on the views of right and wrong held by other people. During the latency period, girls are often physically and intellectually more advanced than boys, and show more emotional stability.

At puberty there is a rapid spurt of growth and physical development and the secondary sexual characteristics make their appearance. A stable young person in understanding surroundings will usually be able to cope with the difficulties posed by all this physical and emotional change, but even the most normal adolescent tends to be moody, unpredictable and even rebellious at times. The physical and emotional aspects of maturation are often temporarily out of step, particularly in modern times when there is such rapid physical development. Society's pressures are sometimes conflicting, since at one moment it treats the adolescent as a child and at another as an adult. The adolescent himself is confused by the alternation between his dependence on his parents and his desire to be free of all supervision. There is often a brief phase of intense friendships during which the girl may develop "crushes" on women whom she admires and the boy goes through a stage of hero-worship. Then there is normally a rapidly awakening interest in the opposite sex. This may lead to some degree of sexual experimentation, but if this is not possible there may be a good deal of masturbation which often leads to feelings of anxiety and guilt (see page 149). There is frequently greater or lesser difficulty in fitting into the more adult type of sexual role and in being at ease in mixed company.

Most adolescents pass through this stage reasonably well and make a satisfactory adjustment to society at the end of it. But adolescence is a time for the re-awakening of emotional conflicts and the possibilities of maladjustment are legion. The young person who is especially immature, who is lacking in drive or whose initiative is stifled by adults may fail to surmount the various obstacles and as a result is likely to remain emotionally retarded. This can cause difficulties in the sexual sphere or may result in more generalized disorders of the personality which interfere with efficient social functioning.

The healthy young person usually maintains a variety of interests and has a good grip on reality. When he has cleared the hurdle of adolescence he enters the stage of young adulthood. During this time he may undergo some form of vocational training, become a wage earner or even get married. The well-balanced individual is able to fit into each of these roles and does not have great difficulty in adjusting from one to the other. As time goes on there are further adjustments to make, this time to parenthood, promotion at work, change of workplace and of habitation, to the making of new friends and the taking up of new interests and activities. The modern woman is no longer tied to the home and to her children as her mother once was, and increased freedom means that she too has to contend with a greater number of social situations and problems.

Nowadays, middle age is regarded with much less foreboding than previously. Certainly it marks the end of the woman's reproductive capacity, but if she can accept this change it often means that her social activities are considerably widened. There is no sudden signpost of middle age in men equivalent to the woman's menopause, but at the present time the rates for illness and death in men rise very sharply during their forties and fifties. This leads to a good deal of widowhood as women on the whole outlive their husbands. However, the majority of people can expect to go on leading active and productive lives till well into their sixties when, of course, the adjustment to retirement must be made. Provided the old person retains good physical health and has kept up some kind of interest, he or she can remain happy and socially active to an advanced age, even though this is a period of gradual diminution of intellectual and emotional capacity during which life is gently slowing down. Contrary to general belief, old people are not usually morbidly preoccupied with impending death unless they are suffering from a good deal of physical or mental illness.

The Material Environment

After birth, the child's mother constitutes the greater part of the environment as he perceives it and in earliest infancy he responds to mother in a totally self-interested way. The very young infant gives pleasure to mother mainly because the normal woman is made in such a way that she gladly gives in to his demands. As time passes and his environment expands he learns to modify these demands, and if you like, he begins to live by the reality principle rather than by the pleasure principle. The material environment is just as important to his emotional development as it is to his physical development. Obviously, nutrition is a basic need and without adequate food he will fail to develop physically. If he survives to adulthood this will lead not only to physical stunting but also to intellectual and emotional impairment. The socioeconomic group to which he belongs will have a marked influence on nutritional and housing standards and will determine to some extent the patterns of illness from which he will suffer throughout life. It will also have an effect on his intelligence and attainment levels and the opportunities he may have to realize his talents.

The environment also has more subtle effects. If a child is brought up in the sort of background where he receives no intellectual encouragement, or where his social contacts are greatly restricted, he is unlikely to achieve anything like the full potential of his intelligence or personality. A poor home and an over-large family often mean that a child has little individual contact with his parents and there is no premium on education or on the need to bring out his particular qualities. This deprivation effect may be seen in even more extreme form in children who spend prolonged periods in the poorer type of orphanage or other form of institution and who have little or no contact with adults or with advantageous environmental stimuli. These children not uncommonly show quite marked emotional and intellectual retardation.

Interpersonal Relationships and Their Importance to the Developing Personality

The structure of the family and the influences which the family brings to bear upon the individual vary widely according to time, place and social class, among other factors. In our present-day society the family tends to be a somewhat isolated unit, usually consisting of parents and children alone and having minimal contact with other generations. We are a mobile society and we often change locality before an opportunity has arisen for prolonged personal relationships to flourish outside the family. Families are, on average, smaller than they used to be so that the relationship between parents and children is often more intense nowadays though discipline has become much less severe. With the frequent emphasis on prolonged education and training, children often remain tied to the parental home for a very long time. All these factors make for heightened intensity of the relationships between individual members of a family and a good deal of one-to-one dependence.

The Western pattern of family structure is certainly not typical of all other societies and even within our own community we can discern many different approaches to child-rearing. Many cultures retain the extended family structure where several generations continue to live under one roof and where relationships are wider and perhaps somewhat less intense from individual to individual. The single human being counts for rather less and a child may be dependent on several adults instead of on just one or two. This type of environment is often fairly conservative and intellectual stimulation may be relatively lacking, but the network of emotional relationships can be very supportive.

In other places, child-rearing goes to the other extreme and there is an insistence on the child's being separated from his parents so that he can be trained in a particular way from an early age. Ancient Sparta was a pathological example of this form of upbringing since parent–child relationships were actively discouraged and children were trained for war from their earliest years. Our society practises a lesser form of this type of child-raising when it sends young children to boarding-school. In Israel, children brought up in a Kibbutz are separated from their parents during the day but see them in the evenings and, to counter any possible ill-effects from such separation, a great deal of emphasis is laid on the need for showing emotional warmth towards these children.

Some societies place a high value on permissiveness while others are very authoritarian in their approach to the rearing of the child. No matter what form the upbringing takes or how extreme it has been, the majority of young people who emerge at the end of it possess recognizably human personalities, which demonstrates how resilient the developing personality is. Yet each person is different from his neighbour and these differences are the result of hereditary and environmental influences and the interplay between them. As well as this, every society contains a proportion of people who are psychologically disturbed and reports that there are cultures which are free of mental illness are mostly to be taken with a pinch of salt. A great deal of argument still goes on as to whether genetic or environmental influences are responsible for mental illness, and among the latter, faulty upbringing has frequently been cited as a cause of various disorders. In fact we have no proof that severe psychotic illnesses like manic-depressive illness and schizophrenia vary much in frequency from country to country and we would expect striking national differences if upbringing had much to do with their actual causation. There is more likelihood that the incidence of psychoneurosis could be increased by adverse early life experiences and there is little doubt that a severely disturbed early life or a childhood home which does not provide adequate emotional support is associated with the causation of personality disorders and especially psychopathy.

Numerous dogmatic statements may be found in the literature regarding the influence of upbringing on the developing personality and on the predisposition to mental illness. For example, it has been suggested that Western culture, with its close relationship between parent and child, is particularly conducive to superego development, while primitive societies, with their lower emphasis on the individual, do not allow the superego to develop fully. This view has been used to explain why there is a proliferation of taboos in certain cultures, since these can be regarded as a means of protecting the community when individual consciences are ineffectual. Modern society does still hold to certain taboos (for example, that against incest) but they are a good deal less formalized and unbreakable than they are amongst many primitive people. There is a great deal of this sort to be learned from intercultural studies as regards the manifestations of psychiatric illness and the ways in which these can be modified by differences of personality structure but we do not know enough about these subjects to be dogmatic. It is therefore necessary for the time being to regard the type of theory we have just mentioned as being purely hypothetical, though it has a great deal of intrinsic interest.

The Function of the Family in Personality Development

A human infant is so helpless that it obviously cannot survive on its own, but it is not just material care and comfort that it requires. The family provides most of the stimulation and emotional warmth that the young child needs for normal psychological development. A stable family environment provides a degree of consistency which is very necessary to him and it also provides a safe ground wherein he can practise new-found skills, learn to cope with strange situations and find out what constitutes the limits of acceptable behaviour. As we have indicated, the initial presence of a mother-figure (who need not be the real mother) is vital because her care and attention provide the earliest form of communication with the child. There is no inherently mysterious bond between mother and infant, though the natural mother is more likely to love her child and so treat it better than someone else would. So far as may be judged, there are no infallible rules which the mother should observe in caring for her infant. It is her general attitude which matters more than any particular practice she may indulge in.

Emotional Deprivation in Early Life

On occasions, a mother may be unable to display a proper maternal attitude towards her infant. There may be various reasons for this: for example, the mother may be brusque and masculine in her outlook or she may be an aloof individual, or she may be too immature herself to feel adequate emotion towards the child. If this situation is not corrected the child may develop symptoms due to emotional deprivation and in the more severe cases this may give rise to quite marked personality disturbances, though it usually takes a fairly profound degree of deprivation to produce abnormalities of this type. It is often taught that any separation of a mother and a young child is to be avoided, but many of the fears about the effects of short-term separation have been ill-founded. Nowadays it is coming to be accepted that separation of itself is not especially damaging, provided the child can relate adequately to a substitute parent-figure. The danger with separation is that a surrogate parent may not be available at the time and then the child may be left in an emotional vacuum at a stage when it has a profound need for security and care. This danger is greatest during the earliest years of life. It is often assumed that it is only loss of the mother which is harmful but it appears that loss of the father or having an inadequate father-figure may be a factor of some significance in the genesis of at least psychopathy and delinquency. Emotional deprivation may also occur when there is neglect or cruelty, even when no separation has occurred, and this may indeed be a more important source of psychological disorder than actual loss of a parent in our society.

Intellectual Maturation

At birth, the infant has very few aptitudes and most of the abilities he will display at a later stage have to be learned. The brain-structures which form the organic basis of mind have already been formed but are still very immature. Within these structures are generated the physico–chemical reactions which are ultimately translated into emotion and thought, but before these reactions become meaningful a long process of learning has to be undergone. Environment is extremely significant in evoking the child's inborn potential: even by the time of birth the intellectual capacity may have been adversely affected by an inadequate intra-uterine nutritional level or by brain-damage during delivery. Thereafter, the material environment and the degree of intellectual stimulation which the child experiences will be largely responsible for the manner in which the intelligence potential is realized.

In earliest infancy, some children are obviously more alert and are quicker to learn than others. They pass their various milestones sooner and they are able to read and to perform other intellectual tasks at a relatively early age. These children are said to be more intelligent than average and as they become older they usually show a greater ability to think in abstract concepts and to carry out tasks of a problem-solving nature. Nowadays society tends to put a particular premium on high intelligence but it is, in fact, just one facet of the total personality. It is not uncommon for an individual to be extremely intelligent but to have very little motivation, and in the long run his performance may be much poorer than that of a person who is less intelligent but who consistently strives very hard.

There are various tests of intelligence which are widely used to measure the intellectual abilities of children and adults. A reliable test can provide a good estimate of intellectual capacity and it is possible to refine and modify test procedures to ascertain whether an individual is realizing his full potential or whether he is falling below his habitual performance level. To some extent it is also possible to differentiate between innate and acquired ability. However, it is much more difficult to test the factors which determine how efficiently the intelligence is employed; factors such as the degree of intellectual curiosity, the level of aspiration and so on. The Intelligence Quotient is a good general indicator of ability but it is not unfailingly accurate and it may be strongly influenced by cultural factors. In addition, the I.Q. is not the immutable entity many people believe it to be since serial testing may show quite remarkable increases or decreases in intellectual efficiency under certain conditions.

Intelligence is not a unitary faculty. It is a collection of different talents, though there is probably an underlying core of general intellectual ability. The person who is highly intelligent is often widely gifted but in addition he may show a tendency to be talented in some particular field. In order that the intellect may be used most efficiently there has to be access to a reliable memory. Co-ordination is also very important, since alertness and the speedy analysis of information are vital. These factors are partly innate but they can be encouraged by a stimulating environment and by skilled and interest-provoking teaching.

As with the total personality, intelligence undergoes a process of evolutionary change in step with the individual's general development. The very young child is able to think only in concrete terms and everything has to be related to himself before it is understandable. For example, an infant may reason in the following way: "Rain is wet because it wets me", or "Mummy is nice because she is nice to *me*". Gradually this degree of egocentricity is modified and by the age of puberty the child has usually acquired the ability to think in abstract terms. In terms of sheer intellectual capacity an individual's peak is often reached before the age of 20 and a gradual decline in the ability for creative thinking is obvious after the age of 30 in most people. Fortunately, intellectual ability is also dependent on experience and maturity of judgement and in the majority of cases this more than compensates for the diminution in creativity for a very long time. It is normally only as old age is reached that there is a sharper fall-off in intellectual efficiency, but even then, as we shall describe in Chapter 10, this can be offset by a slower pace of living and by the old person's increasing obsessionalism which enables him to carry out his duties largely by rote.

The Predisposition to Psychiatric Illness

If the child is fortunate in having a normal genetic background; if nutrition, emotional relationships and the intellectual climate have all been favourable; if his physical health is good and if no unduly traumatic incidents have occurred during his early upbringing, then he is very likely to enjoy a good record of mental health during his adult life. However, any of these variables may be adversely affected and one of the results of this may be a psychiatric disorder. We still remain ignorant of the actual causes of most psychiatric illnesses though we often know why certain phenomena appear in particular conditions. Thus, we cannot explain why it is that only a minority of deprived children go on to develop personality disorders, but we can relate the symptoms in this disturbed minority to the form the deprivation took, the age at which it occurred, and so on.

In subsequent chapters we shall discuss theories of causation of the different psychiatric disorders, but here we would like to introduce some general concepts relating to the aetiology of mental illness. Most psychological theories on this subject introduce the idea of *Conflict* as the keystone of their explanations. If an individual is unable to cope adequately with a problem, emotional conflicts may arise within him as his personality defences struggle to right the situation. If these defences break down, the conflicts become overt and he is said to be suffering from an illness. Some conflicts are almost completely intrapsychic until the defences crumble, whereas others represent a struggle between the individual and his external environment. The particular illness which appears may depend to some extent on the degree of immaturity of the personality and on the particular ego-defences which are called into play. Sometimes the illness as we see it is really the over-emphasis of a defence mechanism. At other times it is a manifestation of a breakdown in all the defences.

Freud's theories are still widely used in explaining these pheno-mena and we shall discuss them briefly, while stressing that they by no means represent proven fact. They have been of greatest service in clarifying certain aetiological aspects of the psychoneurotic illnesses, but, in general, have been quite unsatisfactory when attempting to explain the causes of the more severe psychotic conditions. Freud regarded psychoneurosis as a disturbance of ego-function. Originally, the neurotic symptom is a form of substitute gratification which allows a forbidden thought or deed to be acted out in fantasy. This is a perfectly normal process which at first may be a moderately satisfying substitute for the real thing (viz., daydreaming), but it is never completely successful and there is always a certain amount of frustration. If this form of gratification is sought too often, the frustration will mount and will add to the original state of tension. This, in turn, heightens the need so that there is an ever-diminishing return. All the time, anxiety is growing and when it becomes severe the personality's defences can no longer contain it. When this stage has been reached, the mechanism which once provided gratification has now become a psychological burden and the antagonism between its tension-relieving and its tension-inducing aspects may cause a great deal of "neurotic conflict". We all suffer from some degree of neurotic conflict and it is only when it gets out of control that we can regard the person as being ill.

Every child has to learn to repress emotion in order to gain a realistic amount of control over his instinctual impulses. For one reason or another over-repression may occur, and this has the effect of reducing the available amount of "ego energy" which can be used as the "fuel" for the individual's emotional life. If repression is severe and widespread in the personality, there may be very little free emotional energy left and everyday living then becomes very difficult. Every little event assumes the proportions of a crisis and the person's habitual reaction becomes one of severe anxiety.

Most psychoneurotic illnesses contain this element of pathological anxiety and in the condition known as "Anxiety Neurosis" it is the main symptom. Psychodynamically this illness is interpreted as being due to repression of unacceptable hostile impulses and the anxiety represents a primitive fear of retaliation for these impulses. In other forms of psychoneurosis anxiety is almost invariably present, but it is partly disguised or modified by symptoms which have arisen from the predominant ego defence which has been employed. For example, in phobic illness the individual has an unreasonable fear of certain objects or situations, and this indicates that regression has occurred to a reaction which is much more typical of childhood than of adult life. In many cases the phobia appears to develop because the person is unable to face some problem in the here-and-now, often because the problem contains overtones of unwelcome sexuality. In hysteria, repression and denial are the most notable mechanisms of defence, and here they are being used to protect the patient against adult emotional relationships with which she is unable to cope but from which she is unable to extricate herself. Her anxiety may be converted to a variety of other symptoms, some psychological and some physical. In addition, the hysterical patient often appears to obtain a certain amount of gratification or gain from the illness itself. The obsessive-compulsive individual defends himself from ego-alien impulses by performing rituals which possess an almost magical quality. They prevent anxiety while he is performing them and by their performance he may convince himself for a time, as a child does, that he has undone the harm he imagines has been caused by the impulses.

The behaviour disorders and personality disorders are conditions which are usually present from an early age and which are characterized by persistently abnormal behaviour. In individuals with these disorders there is a good deal of acting-out behaviour and it would seem that, whereas the neurotic represses his conflicts, the individual with a personality disorder allows his to be expressed overtly. However, the process is not always complete and many of these people also have neurotic complaints. In a rather similar way the various sexual disorders are sometimes said to be a "substitute for neurosis" and the forms which they assume appear to be mainly determined by the stage of maturity at which emotional development was halted for one reason or another.

In depressive illness the emotions are turned in on the individual instead of being overtly expressed and the patient experiences a great deal of guilt and self-deprecation. Self-destructive urges are not uncommon and may lead to suicidal behaviour. Because depressive symptoms have a marked similarity to the manifestations of mourning it has been postulated that the illness is really a symbolic form of grief in which the patient mourns for a lost love-object. The loss gives rise to aggressive feelings as well as grief because the patient equates loss with desertion, but this aggression is unthinkable in the circumstances and has to be turned inwards instead of gaining expression.

All of these psychodynamic formulations are valuable in enabling us to interpret the phenomena of psychiatric illness, but, as we have indicated, they do not really tell us about basic causes. They lay a good deal of stress on the importance of environmental events, but this must not be allowed to obscure the equal significance of factors such as hereditary abnormalities, brain dysfunction, biochemical disturbances and so on, since these undoubtedly play a part in the aetiology of at least some of the psychiatric conditions with which we have to deal. Modern psychiatry acknowledges the probable validity of many psychodynamic theories, but it is no longer widely believed that they constitute a comprehensive system of medical psychology.

CHAPTER 4

The Classification and Assessment of Psychiatric Illness

Psychiatry: Fact versus Dogma

Until now we have mostly been describing normal human growth and development although we have pointed out that normal psychological development can be thwarted in a great number of ways at any point in its course and that this may result in various forms of psychiatric illness. In many ways we are still remarkably ignorant of the manner in which this occurs and our theories are at best provisional attempts to clarify an exceedingly complex series of events. Our knowledge of normal psychology is still very incomplete and accurate knowledge about abnormal psychology remains relatively scanty. The psychology of mental illness is a subject of intrinsic fascination, but of course it cannot simply be studied for its academic interest. When we see mental illness we see a patient who is sick and suffering and it should be our aim to increase our knowledge of the subject with the main purpose of decreasing suffering.

There is an unfortunate tendency for psychology and psychiatry to be ideological battlefields on which opposing groups of theoreticians, clinging stubbornly to their own beliefs, do their best to beat down the opposition. This type of argument is not only unprofessional and unscientific, it is potentially harmful to the patient. Time spent quarrelling would be better spent carrying out research to obtain accurate and verifiable data about psychiatric illness. Psychiatry is greatly in need of scientific knowledge: be prepared to accept that much of our present information is useful in providing a framework within which we can work when treating our patients, but never be persuaded that it is revealed truth. Do not be surprised or upset if your knowledge of psychiatry appears to become rapidly out of date. So far as psychiatry is concerned this is a healthy sign because the discipline is developing rapidly in many ways and it suggests an inflexibility of outlook if one cannot accept such change.

There has always been an undue tendency in psychiatry to accept hypothesis as proven fact and to accept observation as explanation. Psychiatry as a scientific study is a relatively young subject and it is still busy describing and classifying illness, a stage that general medicine passed many years ago. Treatment remains largely on an empirical basis and when it is successful we have only the beginnings of insight into why this is so. A great deal of hypothesizing goes on, some of it quite ludicrous, and many psychiatrists still find it easier to conjure up a new theory than to do a worthwhile piece of research. Many people (and not only psychiatrists) find it easier still to be totally unadventurous and stick to the old theories even though these no longer square with up-to-date information.

By means of careful observation it has been possible to see how, in some psychiatric patients, normal mental processes come to be used abnormally and how in others intrinsically abnormal processes may appear. We can also observe how certain symptoms tend to cluster together in a particular way to form recognizable illnesses. Unfortunately, simple observation rarely tells us *why* these things are happening so we have to devise theories in an attempt to explain the phenomena. But these theories should not just be dreamed up: they should be based on previous knowledge and they should be testable to see whether they agree with facts and whether they enable us to predict accurately the outcome of certain events. As a simple example, we might say that it is our theory that a particular drug will cure depression. We know from experience the symptoms which constitute depression and the course the illness is likely to follow without treatment, so by giving the drug we can tell whether a cure has been effected and the theory vindicated. The theory is even more striking if the drug has never been used to treat depression before, but has been chosen because its chemical formula suggests that it should have an antidepressant effect. This is of course a very restricted theory, but in psychiatry there are still very few reliable general theories.

Fortunately, although our knowledge of cause and effect in psychiatric illness is still very scanty, the efficacy of our treatments has improved greatly in recent years, and we are now able to be much more optimistic about the outcome of many psychiatric conditions. A wide range of therapies has become available and more and more of these can be tailored to suit the individual patient. Many lay people are still afraid of psychiatry and regard it as a kind of black magic. They feel that somehow it is dehumanizing to tinker with an individual's mind. We would reply that we are no longer tinkering and that, in any case, it is much more dehumanizing to have to suffer from the illnesses which the psychiatrist and his colleagues are trying to cure. Psychiatry is mostly a rather prosaic and matter-of-fact subject which may disappoint those who are looking for some form of mystical experience. It is at its most effective when it eschews drama and mystery, but we believe that matter-of-factness can always be accompanied by sympathy and human warmth.

The Classification of Psychiatric Illnesses

The needs of patients with different psychiatric conditions vary widely: in order to help these people most effectively and in order to plan our services most efficiently we must have a reliable system of diagnosis. In this chapter we present a classificatory schema which follows the traditional pattern to be found in most textbooks, but we have considerably simplified it for the benefit of the non-psychiatrist.

    1. *Psychoneurosis*
        A. Anxiety state
        B. Depressive reaction (neurotic depression)
        C. Obsessional neurosis
        D. Phobic state
        E. Hysteria

2. *Personality disorders*

    A. A number of conditions resembling the various psychoneurotic conditions (above) but usually beginning at a relatively early age and remaining more or less habitual. These are often associated with some degree of personality inadequacy

    B. Psychopathy
        (i) Inadequate
        (ii) Aggressive
        (iii) Creative

    C. Sexual deviations (including homosexuality, lesbianism, sado-masochism, voyeurism, exhibitionism, etc.)

3. *Alcoholism* ⎤ These conditions frequently complicate pre-
4. *Drug addiction* ⎦ existing personality disorders

5. *Psychosis*

    A. Organic
        (i) Acute (delirium)
        (ii) Chronic (dementia)
        (iii) Miscellaneous conditions including personality changes due to brain-damage and chronic epilepsy

    B. Functional
        (i) Affective disorders (various types of depression, mania, some forms of anxiety)
        (ii) Schizophrenic states (simple, hebephrenic, catatonic, paranoid)
        (iii) Others (including certain rather rare paranoid states and atypical familial psychoses)

6. *Suicide and attempted suicide*

7. *Mental subnormality* ⎤ Not dealt with in this volume as they
8. *Child psychiatry* ⎦ are sufficiently complex subjects to require separate treatment

While it is possible to categorize psychiatric illness as we have just done, it must be admitted that in practice it is often a good deal more difficult to assign a particular case to its diagnostic niche. In many instances the patient has symptoms suggestive of more than one type of illness, or else the symptoms are so profoundly altered by personality characteristics or environmental influences that it is difficult to distinguish the underlying illness. A disorder may alter in appearance very considerably according to the stage of its progress and the initial diagnosis may have to be changed more than once: for example, a schizophrenic illness can present as a typical psychoneurosis at the outset, then go through a phase closely resembling manic-depressive illness and only develop the unmistakable features of schizophrenia at a relatively late stage. Thereafter, if the illness is halted before it becomes unduly severe it may have many of the appearances of a personality disorder.

In psychiatric illnesses which are due to organic disease it may be possible to demonstrate objectively the cause of the disorder: in a case of epilepsy there may be a piece of scar tissue in the brain which is initiating the seizures, in dementia it may be possible to demonstrate on X-ray that the brain has become atrophic, and in some cases of delirium it may be shown that the mental abnormality is due to a temporary accumulation of toxic products in the blood owing to liver or kidney failure. Nowadays by far the greater number of psychiatric cases are not due to organic disease and these show no objectively verifiable aetiological abnormalities. Therefore, in order to make a diagnosis we have to depend on the complaints made by the patient, his behaviour, and the history obtained from him and from his acquaintances. Then, because there is a certain amount of subjectivity in the process, the diagnostic formulation will depend to some extent on the psychiatrist's experience and theoretical outlook. This makes for a somewhat unsatisfactory situation and it may be asked why we bother to make a detailed diagnosis at all. The answer to this is that if one does not have a classificatory system every patient becomes a unique problem and there is no real opportunity of comparing the effects of treatment in different types of illness in order to find which treatment is best for which condition. In psychiatry we are prepared to admit that the patient is unique, but not his illness. Psychiatric illnesses do seem to fall into a number of broad categories and the reality of this division appears to be confirmed by the tendency of each group to respond differently to treatment. However, there is no cause for complacency and we must always be prepared to abandon traditional diagnostic criteria if new ones prove more reliable.

Aetiological Factors in Psychiatric Illness

Many people object to the idea that psychiatric disorders can be regarded in much the same way as physical illnesses. Admittedly it is usually more difficult to define and describe a psychiatric condition, but there is no reason to think that it is essentially different in its nature or causation from a physical ailment. Illness of any kind is rarely a simple matter of cause and effect. Only occasionally does a psychiatric condition arise in this way, as for example when a workman drops a brick on the head of an innocent passer-by in the street below, causing brain damage and subsequent dementia. Much more often there is a complex series of circumstances which predispose the individual to illness and precipitate him into it, and this is equally true in both physical and mental disorder. Before we pronounce on the cause of the condition and the way in which we intend to treat it, we have to take all the important variables into account.

It is natural for someone engaged in social work to be particularly interested in the part played by social and environmental factors in the causation of mental illness. Undoubtedly these often do exert a great deal of influence: the patient's upbringing, adverse events which have occurred at various stages in the course of his development, chronic insecurity, lack of proper parental care and supervision, and many other possible traumatic experiences, may have had profoundly disturbing effects on the immature personality. These effects may be opposed by various defence mechanisms but under stress these mechanisms may ultimately give way. The stage of life at which the stress occurs may be important since there are a number of age groups in which breakdown seems more than usually liable to occur. Adolescence is a notably stormy period; engagement and then the responsibilities of being newly married may have adverse effects on some; childbirth and the menopause are associated with mental disorder in a proportion of women; and retirement, old age and bereavement can all produce difficulties of adjustment.

In the individual's current life situation there are possibly many factors which conspire to distress him and perhaps precipitate illness. He may have to cope with insecurities at home because of estranged parents, marital tensions or, in an older generation, inability to see eye-to-eye with the children. Such problems may be short-lived or can be more permanent and they may be due to potentially remediable causes or to clashes of utterly incompatible temperaments. There may be other background tensions such as overcrowding, living in rooms or with parents, and lack of privacy. Poor wages or inability to keep to a budget may well aggravate the situation and are likely to make the patient feel quite hopeless about the possibility of ever getting out of it. Furthermore, these vulnerable people are often the ones who get into debt and lose their employment. Physical ill-health is another important cause of psychological stress—for example, in the young mother who has had too many children too quickly, the middle-aged woman having a stormy passage through the menopause or the old person who is isolated by deafness or blindness.

Other social factors may also have to be considered. The person is perhaps in unsuitable employment, either because he has too much responsibility or because he is anxious to gain promotion but is held to a humbler task because of lack of qualifications. He may simply dislike the work he is doing, or in the case of some married women there may be considerable resentment that they have to work at all when they already have a house and family to look after. Apart from the work there may possibly be considerable interpersonal difficulties which cause tension—for example, bickering with neighbours, quarrelling with relatives and so on.

Any of these environmental variables may be regarded as a possible precipitating factor in psychiatric illness and one of them, or a combination of them, may prove overwhelming to the individual. However, it has to be asked why one person breaks down under a strain of this sort and others manage to cope. Often there is no clear-cut answer to such a question, but one suspects that other factors must be present before a nervous illness occurs and we shall shortly be discussing some of these. It is tempting to attribute the onset of a psychiatric disorder to some event which has occurred immediately before. Certainly when one is taking a history it is necessary to record any circumstances which could have contributed to the illness, but it is best to be cautious when it comes to deciding what were the actual causal factors. Sometimes the apparent cause can actually turn out to be a result of the illness: for example, a patient with an obvious depressive condition may claim that it began as a result of his having been dismissed from work, and this seems a reasonable explanation for his illness. It is only when close enquiry is made that it becomes obvious that his depression has been creeping up on him, unnoticed for a considerable time, and it was its interference with his concentration and efficiency which had brought about his dismissal. At other times, of course, a depression will actually be the result of a traumatic event, but it is usually wise to seek for other predisposing factors as well.

It is always necessary to make enquiry about hereditary and constitutional factors in psychiatric illness since these can sometimes be of considerable significance. In some forms of mental subnormality and in a number of pre-senile dementing illnesses heredity seems to be almost the entire cause of the condition. In depressive psychosis and in schizophrenia there are probably important genetic influences, but these appear to produce a predisposition which requires the intervention of various environmental factors before the predisposition can emerge in the form of the particular illness. Even in some psychoneurotic illnesses there may be an hereditary element: for example, obsessional neurosis often occurs in families where many of the members have marked obsessional traits though it is difficult to be sure if this is due to heredity or particular patterns of upbringing.

There are some physical illnesses which appear to have an association with mental disorder. One of these is essential hypertension, a form of raised blood pressure which often appears in various members of the same family and probably has a genetic basis in many cases: individuals with this condition appear excessively liable to develop depressive disorders and in a case of depression it is always wise for the doctor to check the blood pressure. In schizophrenia certain constitutional abnormalities tend to occur to excess: these patients frequently have cold, blue hands and feet, rather low blood pressure and excessively greasy skin. Apart from physical illness it would appear that certain normal constitutional features may also have a connection with mental illness and body-build is an example of this. Manic-depressive illness is probably commoner in those of a stocky (pyknic) build whereas schizophrenia is found more often in people with a thin and somewhat droopy physique (the asthenic type). Hysterical illnesses are quite often found in individuals with marked immaturity of physical development. Body-build and personality type often seem to go hand-in-hand, the pyknic individual tending to be more out-going and sociable and the asthenic more withdrawn and solitary: this of course is a generalization and is certainly not universally true. The type of personality often seems able to influence the course of a mental illness and it is usually said that if an individual with a pyknic physique and extroverted personality develops schizophrenia the chance of recovery is much better for him than it is for the introverted, asthenic individual who develops a similar condition.

A number of other physical factors may be important in predisposing to mental illness and the psychiatrist always makes enquiry about the possibility of these having been present when he is assessing a case. Brain damage at birth is incriminated in some cases of mental deficiency and epilepsy and even in some cases of personality disorder where there is evidence of unstable cerebral function. The ordinary infectious diseases of childhood, if they occur with particular severity, may leave the young person habitually nervous and in a small number of cases they may actually cause brain damage in the form of encephalitis (inflammation of the brain). Brain damage can occur in many other ways and at any time of life, by head injury, disease, interference with the brain's blood supply by hardening of the cerebral arteries, and so on. If the damage is severe the usual result is dementia: if it is less severe it may leave a degree of instability which renders the patient more likely to develop other forms of psychiatric disorder. Chronic alcoholism is often a result of some personality disorder but it can, in its turn, produce further symptoms as a result of chronic intoxication, and brain damage due to vitamin deficiency.

It should be mentioned that females are generally more likely than males to break down into psychiatric illness and it has been suggested that this is partly because they are subjected to a good deal of hormonal stress. Each month they undergo a complex series of hormonal changes due to the menstrual cycle and in many women these changes have a marked effect on their mood-state. In some females, pre-menstrual tension can be so severe that it will precipitate a mental illness. Childbearing is also associated with numerous endocrine and other physical changes and a proportion of women who have recently given birth to a child develop puerperal psychosis (see p. 234).

Up till now we have been implying that the way of life can have a profound influence on the prevailing mood-state and on the liability to develop psychiatric illness. The opposite is also true that psychiatric illness can markedly affect the individual's way of life. Obviously the person who is ill may have to stay off work or even go to hospital and these constitute changes in his life-pattern, but in most psychiatric disorders nowadays these are very transitory interruptions in his career. However, in some chronic illnesses the whole pattern of life may be disrupted and this is often found in schizophrenia. It is now well known that this illness undoubtedly tends to be commoner in individuals in the lowest socio-economic strata of society and in those who live in particularly isolated and unsatisfactory circumstances. At first it was thought that poverty and loneliness were the causes of schizophrenia, but now there is much evidence to suggest that it is actually the onset of the illness which in many cases produces a falling-off in the patient's capabilities and a decline in his social status, so that by the time the condition is recognized he has become indigent. Here again we would underline the need for caution in attributing an illness to a particular cause when it is really the result of many interacting influences. It is very tempting, when one has discovered that individuals in some particular section of society display a peculiar pattern of disease-proneness, to infer that special hardships in their way of life have precipitated these diseases. Immigrant populations often show a high rate of mental disorders and it seems logical to assume that the stress of moving from one way of life to another has caused the breakdown. In fact there is evidence that a relatively high proportion of emigrants are unhappy and unstable people who leave home because of excessive restlessness and who would probably break down eventually no matter where they were. This factor of self-selection is sometimes very important in producing a concentration of cases of psychiatric illness in, for example, certain occupations. Highly dangerous tasks are usually associated with a high injury rate, but this injury rate is often greater than it need be because the type of work tends to attract individuals who are reckless and lacking in foresight: in addition, high wages often lead to heavy consumption of alcohol which further increases the accident rate. Thus the rate of physical and mental breakdown in certain occupations is high, partly because the conditions are bad but partly also because of the type of person engaged in the work.

It should be obvious that in order to make a psychiatric assessment a great deal of information must be collected and collated. Once this has been done the process of weighing a series of probabilities begins. For example, what is the likely diagnosis? What were the probable precipitating factors? Can these factors be remedied in order to prevent a recurrence? What is the most suitable treatment? What is the chance of complete recovery? One is most likely to discover accurate answers to these questions if one has enquired into all the possibly relevant factors. The social worker can be invaluable in gathering information which complements and adds to the psychiatric history, and which enables the clinician to make a more accurate and comprehensive assessment of the mental state. We shall now proceed to discuss in some detail the techniques of case-history taking which the social worker will need in order to provide information in the most relevant fashion.

Case-history Taking for the Social Worker

From what we have just said it will be obvious that we regard the case history as a most important element in the process of understanding the patient and his illness. From the point of view of making a psychiatric diagnosis it is not always necessary to have a long and complicated account of the life history but the diagnostic function of the case history is only one of its aspects. Before a prognosis can be formulated (that is, a prediction of the probable course the illness will take and the possibility of recovery) a knowledge of the mode of onset and the progress to date of the illness is vital. Indeed, it is sometimes more valuable in the field of psychiatry to consider illnesses as a series of processes rather than as disease entities: by doing this we can gather information in a more logical manner, though eventually it will be necessary to integrate our data into diagnostic form since this is the first step in planning treatment. The next step, that of prognosis, is equally important and must be based, like the diagnosis, on factual rather than anecdotal case material. As we have seen, treatment in psychiatry is not solely concerned with the patient. It is concerned with the patient in his total environment which includes his family, his home, his work and all the other areas of his existence which affect his psychological well-being. It is extremely important that the mentally sick individual's altered behaviour be viewed with understanding by those around him, and it is part of the social worker's task to see that this happens. However, before we can make any plans to do this it is necessary to learn a great deal about the patient's social constellation. How well do the relatives understand the situation? How much have they been involved in the development of his illness? What kind of support are they capable of providing for the patient during and after treatment?

All these factors and many more make it imperative that facts and observations be collected in detail so that they can be presented in a form which will enable easy comparison to be made between the history given by the patient (which will usually be recorded by the psychiatrist) and that taken by the social worker from a relative or key informant. As we have already shown, without this confirmatory history the process of the illness and its social complications can easily be confused. Though we shall present a method of history taking and suggest those topic-headings which will ensure that all the vital areas are adequately covered, it must be emphasized that the art of efficient history taking can only be achieved through experience and by taking especial pains with the histories one obtains from one's early cases. With experience you may learn to take some short cuts, but do not be tempted to do this during the process of learning.

We have indicated that the case history should be orderly and should follow a pattern, but the system we shall outline need not necessarily be followed in a slavish fashion. The order in which the different topics are discussed with a patient or relative will often be determined largely by the trend the conversation takes. Generally speaking, data should be collected in the most convenient way and later put into a form which will render the information most readily available. It is normally necessary to have several interviews with a patient or relative in order to complete the schema although, in the particular case of patients who have attempted suicide, it is necessary to obtain a detailed case history with the minimum of delay. (Later we shall discuss the additional data which it is helpful to acquire in these cases.)

The great majority of patients are prepared to co-operate in the giving of a detailed account of their lives, but since it is normally the psychiatrist who will gather that information we shall deal largely with case histories taken by social workers from relatives who may be rather less willing to give personal information about the patient. They may sometimes feel it is disloyal or downright wrong to discuss the individual's private life and they may well be reluctant to talk about their own private affairs for a variety of reasons, the commonest being that they cannot understand the necessity for doing so. In many instances they would prefer not to be made aware of any part that they might have played in the genesis of the patient's illness and they do not necessarily assume, as the patient can do with his doctor, that they will enjoy complete confidentiality. The patient, in his interview with the psychiatrist, usually accepts that notes will be taken but the relative who is being interviewed by the social worker may not be at all happy about this.

Note Taking, the Interview and Confidentiality

There is considerable controversy over whether note taking should be carried out during the interview or should be postponed until immediately after it has ended. One school of thought on the subject is against note taking during the interview because it is considered that it tends to hold up the proceedings, may interrupt the social worker's train of thought and may make the patient or relative unduly aware that whatever he is saying is being "taken down in evidence". The other school regards note taking as a convenient and unembarrassing activity on the part of the interviewer while he waits for the informant to express himself. We do not wish to be dogmatic on the subject but we would suggest that, however the interview is conducted, it should have only one end in view and that is to get (at least in the history-taking portion) as much relevant information as possible. Much will depend on the personal preference of the interviewer and the attitude of the interviewee, but the former must be prepared to be flexible and to adjust his method to the particular situation. In general we believe that it is advisable for the interview to be started informally and without any note taking. Some form of free conversation is useful initially because it encourages the informant to relax, it allows the interviewer to decide whether note taking will be permissible and it provides an opportunity to give some reassurance to the informant about his own feelings and about the confidential nature of the interview. Also, it allows the social worker to explain the part she plays in the therapeutic team so that the individual will know from the outset that the information he gives will be made available to the members of the team who will play a part in treatment.

Even if it is thought in a particular case that notes can be taken during interview it is still as well to be aware that, even though adequate reassurances have been given regarding confidentiality, a relative may require further assurances during the session. Sometimes the informant withholds material because he is afraid that the patient might be told what has been said, but if the interview has been successfully conducted in a friendly, tactful and non-critical manner he can be shown that his contribution is not just tale-telling. If he appreciates this he will rarely refuse permission for his information to be discussed with the patient if this happens to be necessary. The skilful interviewer can encourage the patient or relative by acknowledging that what they have to say is important, often important enough to write down there and then. Even the most suspicious relatives will, if they are handled properly, usually end by telling the interviewer directly how they feel about being questioned and especially about note taking. It is not uncommon for the social worker to be told, "Perhaps you should make a note of this", or "I hope you won't forget to tell the doctor that".

Whether or not notes have been taken during interview a period of free discussion towards the end of the session can be valuable to the social worker and helpful to the interviewee. This can perhaps be introduced by telling the informant how helpful he has been and by asking him whether there are any questions he would like answered. The person then often raises queries about the interview itself so this means that the social worker should refrain from asking questions which she is not prepared to explain later in lay terms if the individual wants to know why they were asked. Inviting questions from the informant increases his sense of participation and has the added advantage that it allows him to express his own areas of anxiety which may be vital information for the social worker who will later be working with the patient and perhaps his family as well. One note of caution is worth while making here and that is that one should not be led into expressing too many opinions at this stage. Naturally the relative is usually anxious over the patient's state of health and may ask many leading questions about what he himself should have done in the past or do in the future. Do not be tempted to give specific answers unless you have consulted closely with your medical colleagues and a course of action has been decided.

On the whole it has been found best to leave purely factual questions and questions which may cause some anxiety till near the end of the interview so that before these topics are embarked upon the relative will have had a chance to gain confidence in the social worker and to be reassured that he is providing material which will be of great benefit to the patient.

If note taking is obviously undesirable when a particular informant is present there should be no delay between the interview and its recording. Experiments on "memorizing" clearly indicate that even a short lapse of time gives scope for the interviewer's own unconscious attitudes to distort his record of what has been said. Moreover, from a practical point of view, post-interview note taking can be difficult since time often must elapse between leaving the patient's home (where much social work history taking is carried out) and arriving at the place where the writing can be done. It becomes even more difficult when, because of heavy case-loads, the case worker has conducted a series of interviews before recording any of them. In these circumstances there is a tendency to confuse different cases or to fill in material by noting what one thinks was said rather than what actually was said.

A small but important point is worthy of note here. If the social worker can choose the place where the interview will take place this has the incidental advantage of eliciting unobtrusively the lengths to which a relative or key-person will go in order to help the patient.

Unless there is some great urgency it should be remembered that a series of interviews tends to produce more valuable information because of the growth of confidence between the caseworker and the informant. It should always be a rule that, except in cases where there must be a rapid collection of information (as with attempted suicide, see p. 68), questioning in the face of the informant's hostility should be avoided. It is better to allow him to talk out his aggression and then he will usually see reason because he will find that his hostility does not evoke a similar response.

Some psychiatrists maintain that it is better for them to take the social history themselves, provided that they have the time. There are a number of arguments against this assertion but perhaps the most important is that patients and relatives nearly always ascribe to the psychiatrist the authoritarian role of "doctor" and will tell him only those things which they believe to be important from a medical point of view. On the other hand, when they get to know the social worker's role and the purpose of her work they can often confide to her all the environmental circumstances which might otherwise be overlooked or be considered as unworthy for a doctor's ears! It is necessary in the patient's best interests for the information gathered by the psychiatrist and the social worker to be amalgamated so that the illness may be understood in its appropriate context and in order that treatment can be realistically directed according to the internal and external resources of the patient and his family. To this end there should be no sense of rivalry between the two colleagues: it is by their combined skill that the patient will best be helped.

We have mentioned the special need for urgency in the case of attempted suicide. Most psychiatric conditions are of relatively long duration and their onset is comparatively slow. It is therefore usually possible to gather social information over a reasonable period of time in order to gain the maximum of useful material. However, attempted suicide often occurs in the setting of an acute social and psychiatric crisis and its manifestations are analogous in many ways to a medical emergency. In order to obtain an accurate account of the complex precipitating factors, the patient's environmental circumstances and the amount of help otherwise to be expected from the relatives, a social history is necessary straight away. The patient is often admitted to a general hospital for resuscitation and following recovery from the attempt the question of disposal may be an urgent one. The psychiatric team must have the appropriate information as quickly as possible in order to decide on a course of action and in this situation the social worker will be required to produce an adequate history within the shortest possible time. This demands especial skill and tact in order to avoid heightening further an already highly emotional situation in the patient's household.

Setting Out a Social History

1. The history should always be prefaced by the following information: the patient's civil status (that is, whether single, married or other), date of birth, address, the source of referral and the reason for referral to the social worker. The social worker's name should be clearly appended so that she can be contacted by the psychiatrist without undue delay when this is necessary.

2. *Informants*

The name and address of the informant or informants should be recorded, together with their relationship to the patient and some comment as to the circumstances of the interview. It should be noted whether the informants were seen separately or together and there should be an assessment of their reliability as witnesses. The degree of reliability can be affected by, for example, intellectual backwardness, hostility, untruthfulness or simply lack of knowledge of these details which would be of help to the psychiatrist and the social worker. The presence of any such factors should be recorded.

Hereafter, the order in which the history is ascertained, the relative importance attached to particular topics and the need for the addition of special sections will depend very much on the setting in which the social worker is employed and the role which is expected of her by her agency. The format will also be dependent to some extent on the special interests of the psychiatrist in charge of the case, the use made by the hospital or agency of printed forms for history taking and the circumstances in which the history is taken. The schema which follows should be sufficiently comprehensive to allow for most eventualities.

3. *The Patient's Family History*

Paternal grandparents and their family, showing the ordinal position of the patient's father within his own sibship.

Maternal grandparents and their family, showing the ordinal position of the patient's mother within her own sibship.

Any nervous or mental illness occurring in either family should be noted along with details of admission to mental hospital, attempted or completed suicide, epilepsy, alcoholism and any psychosomatic disorders.

Father. Give his age and occupation: if he is dead, note his age at death and the cause of death. Provide a description of his personality, his general state of health, details of any past or present serious illnesses and particulars of any psychiatric disorders from which he may have suffered, with information on whatever hospital or outpatient treatment he has received. Note the quality of the relationship between him and the patient: has it altered radically with the passage of time?

Mother. Information should be collected in very much the same way as for father.

The patient's siblings. A similar account should be obtained of each brother and sister. It is convenient to place the siblings' histories in order of descending age, showing the patient's ordinal position in the family but reserving the full account of his personal history for a separate section which will naturally go into much greater detail.

In the family history section, one should include all the information which has been gathered about the personalities of the family members, their degree of stability or instability, their idiosyncrasies of behaviour and an assessment of their ability to adapt to their particular life-circumstances. This should be presented in such a way that the psychiatrist or any other team member can quickly gain an accurate impression of the family as a whole and the influence it has had on the patient throughout his life. As we have explained previously, the family history is intended to provide information on hereditary and environmental influence, on patterns of family health and illness and on predominant modes of behaviour and interaction.

4. *Home Circumstances*

Under this heading should be described the circumstances which are typical of the patient's current life rather than those which were present in his earlier years. Unless financial hardship is patently a significant factor in the patient's mental disturbance it is not usually necessary for the psychiatrist or the social workers to obtain minute details of family income and expenditure. Instead it is important to know whether the income is adequate and whether it is managed reasonably efficiently. It is always worth knowing accurately about the socio-economic group to which the patient belongs and the extent of his mobility from one social class to another.

Nowadays it is not enough to record the district or municipal ward in which the patient lives as an indicator of his social status. Housing shortages, local authority housing policies and the greatly increased level of social mobility have rendered this quite unreliable as a criterion. Instead it is better to discover whether the patient is suited or unsuited to his home area and whether he and his family are happy to conform to the prevailing standards of the neighbour-hood. For this purpose the social worker should have a considerable knowledge of local occupations, standards and customs and until she has acquired this she is unlikely to be completely satisfactory as a reporter of the more generalized aspects of the patient's environ-ment. This account of the patient in his social milieu is a valuable background to the more detailed information on the patient's emotional environment which the psychiatrist will gather from the patient himself. As well as providing general information the social worker can be of great help in obtaining particulars about the occupants of the patient's home and their relationships with each other. There is always a need for an accurate and factual interpre-tation of the home atmosphere with its various strains, conflicts and jealousies as well as its more positive elements, such as the degree of goodwill in the family and the willingness to accept the patient's psychological abnormalities. We have to be fully aware of all the relevant social factors in the illness situation since in psychiatry it is considered that a social recovery is just as important to a patient as a medical recovery.

If domestic friction is a prominent feature of the home situation it should be reported in this section. An account should be given of how it began and there should be a description of the forms it takes. However, if the friction appears to be related only to the patient's married life, the details would be more appropriately relegated to the section which deals with his personal history.

5. Personal History

The pre-school period. The amount of information which it is appropriate to obtain under this heading will vary greatly according to the age of the patient, the nature of his illness and the knowledge possessed by the informant. In some circumstances (notably in child guidance work) it will be relevant to include information about the condition of the patient's mother during pregnancy, her attitude towards being an expectant mother and details of any complications prior to or during the confinement. Details of the patient's early development are important: for instance, whether he was healthy or delicate, precocious or retarded. The social worker should note when he passed his various childhood milestones such as teething, talking, walking and toilet-training. Particular attention should be paid to indications of neurotic symptoms in childhood, like night-terrors, sleep-walking, temper tantrums, bed-wetting, thumb-sucking, nail-biting, food fads, stammering, behaviour mannerisms and specific or non-specific anxieties.

Pay attention to any outstanding events which occurred to parents or other members of the household during the patient's early years. It is particularly important to discover about any notable episodes of separation from the parents during childhood and to try to assess the patient's reaction to their absence. In addition it is necessary to obtain details of the parent surrogate to find out whether the patient received adequate physical and emotional care when the parents were away.

Make enquiry into the emotional relationships between the patient and his parents, siblings and relatives to discover whether these bonds were stable and happy or disrupted and unsatisfactory.

School. This section will include information on the age at which the patient started school and the length of time his education lasted. Note the standard which was attained and any especial successes or failures. Enquire too about the parental attitudes towards the patient's academic performance and whether this came up to their expectations. Find out whether the patient was happy at school and what sort of relationship he had with his teachers and schoolmates. Did he join in any extracurricular activities? In taking this part of the history the social worker often has to use her critical judgement because patients and their relatives have a habit of describing their school careers in over-optimistic terms.

Play. Here it is appropriate to include details of the patient's ability to get on with other children when he was younger. For example, was he shy and somewhat solitary or did he make friends easily, play games and join youth organizations or societies? During adolescence did he participate in organized games and did he take an active part in the other social activities of his contemporaries?

Employment record. Give a chronological account of the patient's work record since leaving school, noting the reasons given for his changing jobs. Has he been a steady worker, has he shifted from job to job, has he frequently been dismissed? Some intimation should be given of the skill required for his present occupation and whether changes of employment have led to advancement. Be sure to enquire after any feature of his work which appears to have been associated with the onset of his illness. Note if the patient has served in the Armed Forces, and if war service has led to injury; mention this fact here but expand on the details when describing his health record.

Psychosexual development. This is an area of great delicacy which calls for considerable sensitivity and tact on the part of the interviewer. It is important when asking questions about topics which are normally considered to be embarrassing to be as natural in manner as possible, neither too diffident nor too blasé. You must not give the person the impression that you are prying unnecessarily into the more intimate details of the patient's life. Among the matters which you may wish to discuss are adolescent "crushes" on members of the same sex, masturbation and the guilt feelings it frequently engenders, the patient's first sexual experience, his sexual fantasies and the adequacy of his present sexual outlets. You may also want to know the strength of his sex drive and whether it is directed predominantly to his own or the opposite sex. In female patients it is important to obtain some details regarding menstruation and any notable mood-changes which occur during the menstrual cycle. Where appropriate, information about the menopause will be sought. Much of this information is only obtainable from the patient so do not pursue the subject unnecessarily if the relative obviously cannot provide the answers.

Marriage. This section includes information about the courtship and the circumstances of the marriage, including whether it was a forced wedding because the girl had become pregnant. The patient's attitudes towards having children, his general marital relations and any specific sexual difficulties should be noted here. Is there anxiety about the possibility of another pregnancy? Are contraceptive methods used, and if so, does their use give rise to any conflict or anxiety? Again, since many of these are extremely delicate topics the questioning will have to be gentle and, at times, fairly indirect.

The patient's spouse. Deal here with data about the age, the personality and the physical and mental health of the spouse. Describe his or her occupational history and social background. Find out about the attitude towards children and the relationship with the family. It is often valuable to give one's impression of the degree of harmony or otherwise which exists between the couple.

Children. Provide a chronological list of the patient's children, giving their ages, sex and individual names. Make a brief record of their personalities, health and attitudes towards each other and to their parents. Were the children welcome additions to the family and are any more wanted? Have either the patient or the spouse had any miscarriages: if so, how many?

6. *Health*

Under this heading are gathered details of the patient's health record since earliest childhood, giving details and dates of illnesses or accidents and noting whether there were any hospitalizations.

It is also customary to report here on habits which may influence the individual's health, such as the amount of alcohol he drinks and with what frequency, his tobacco consumption and whether he takes drugs of any sort. Information about eating and sleeping patterns is also valuable. Enquiry should always be made as to whether there have been any marked changes in the recent past with regard to habits and health.

7. *Personality*

This is one of the most important parts of the history because it informs the psychiatrist about characteristics which may be quite submerged by the symptoms of the illness. An account should be obtained of the patient's pre-morbid personality to discover what its main features were. Was he moody, restless, excitable, suspicious or was he steady and placid? Was he lacking in initiative, dull and unenthusiastic or was he excessively careful and methodical? Was he adaptable or readily upset when faced with strange situations? Was he a reliable person who could easily cope with responsibility, was he kind, sympathetic and imaginative or was he remote and secretive? Was he an organizer or a follower, was he aggressive or submissive and dependent? Did he usually prefer the company of the same or of the opposite sex? These are the sort of items of information which the social worker will be looking for but it often proves easier to obtain the answers by indirect questioning— for example, by asking how he spent his time, what his interests and hobbies were, whether or not he helped around the house and so on. Relatives can usually answer these sort of questions but may be quite unable to give a satisfactory reply to direct enquiries about particular characteristics.

The patient's normal mood should be described in terms such as cheerful, despondent, anxious or worrying. Did he create an over-all impression of self-satisfaction or self-deprecation, modesty or over-confidence, stability or vacillation, self-control or over-indulgence? Finally, some details should be given about the patient's standards of living, about his moral and religious views and about his practical and social approach to the family's affairs.

8. *Previous Mental Ill-health*

It is important to obtain details of all the psychiatric conditions from which the patient has suffered, even if no treatment has been required. If he has received treatment one should note the form it took and where it was carried out. The approximate date and duration of each episode of illness should be recorded.

Even if there have been no previous attacks of psychiatric illness enquire about the possible existence of such psychological symptoms as hysterical outbursts, preoccupation with bodily functions, complaints of insomnia, mood variations, psychosomatic complaints, obsessional ruminations and excessive anxiety. In addition, take account of any reported character abnormalities (including delinquency) or behaviour disturbances which have been noted by acquaintances though not necessarily by the patient himself.

9. *Present Illness*

This will mainly be the concern of the psychiatrist but it is a considerable help for him to have another person's account of events like the first occurrence of altered behaviour in the patient, impaired social efficiency and pathological changes of mood. It is important too to give details of circumstances which appear to have been associated with the onset of the illness, paying particular attention to dates and times if a causal connection is suspected. As well as finding out what made the relatives suspect that the patient was unwell one should also enquire as to the circumstances which made him unmanageable at home if this has been the case. This last point is of some importance since relatives may require a great deal of reassurance about possibly alarming features of this illness once the patient has recovered and is ready to go home.

10. *Any Other Information*

Quite often it is necessary to have a section of this sort to allow for the inclusion of miscellaneous data. Most information can be recorded under the headings we have suggested, but sometimes we are provided with material which does not conveniently fit into these categories. Rather than be tempted to twist it to fit, or even to forget it altogether, be prepared to note it separately.

The Social Worker's Approach to Case-history Taking

A social history presented in the form which we have outlined may not be studied in its entirety by the psychiatrist, but it should enable him to extract quickly the information which he requires for a full assessment of the case. The remainder of the history should contain data which are useful to the social worker: try to avoid too much redundant material.

Naturally the psychiatrist's tendency will be to make his assessment with a particular emphasis on the medical and psychological aspects of the situation and it is important that the social worker should provide a balance by drawing attention to those social items which appear to have special significance to the illness. To this end we would recommend that each social history should finish with a relatively terse summary of the outstanding points contained in the report, with stress laid by the social worker on those factors which she considers to be of greatest importance.

Throughout this chapter we have laid emphasis on the gathering of factual information. We do not believe that the social worker is simply a clerk who gathers data in a routine and totally unimaginative way. On the contrary, her informed opinion is valuable and will be listened to with respect by the wise psychiatrist. However, her opinion can only be well informed if it is based on accurate records. What the psychiatrist wants is an unvarnished account of what has been told to the social worker together with her skilled observations, free of unnecessary jargon and gratuitous interpretation. You will find that facts usually speak better for themselves than any amount of conjecture.

CHAPTER 5

The Psychoneuroses and Psychosomatic Illnesses

IF YOU were asked to make an estimate of the frequency of mental illness in the community by means of a survey of all the inpatients in psychiatric hospitals at a given time you would probably conclude that (apart from the large problem of mental subnormality) the commonest forms of psychiatric disorder were various types of psychotic illness, dementing conditions (mostly due to old age), personality disorders and a smallish number of psychoneurotics. But this is a very misleading impression since patients in hospitals are mostly those who are most severely ill or whose illnesses are most chronic. Despite the fallacies which are inherent in using hospital admission data, many of our statistics regarding mental illness were, until recently, based on their use.

Nowadays we look much more to the general population for our information and in doing this we produce some surprising results. In the first place we find that psychological disorders are extremely common. No one is quite free from some degree of neurosis, but most of our neurotic fears (such as fear of insects, dislike of heights, aversion to public speaking) are so common as to be socially acceptable. However, at a conservative estimate, about a fifth of the general population is markedly handicapped at some time in life (often for long periods) by psychiatric disorders, and if we include all those people with physical illnesses which appear to have an important emotional component, then the proportion becomes very much higher. The "normal" population in fact contains a high proportion of individuals who have a marked degree of psychological abnormality: by this reckoning it would be abnormal to be psychologically perfect.

Look around any group of human beings and you will find that the majority are coping quite reasonably with everyday life whereas a small minority is almost totally unable to cope. Between these two types is a large number of people who can cope only marginally or intermittently, perhaps because they are physically disabled, mentally retarded, unable to meet the demands of society in some way (for example, criminals), or who are suffering from some form of emotional disorder.

The psychiatrist traditionally distinguishes between the severest forms of mental illness, the *Psychoses,* and the less severe conditions, known as the *Psychoneuroses* or *Neuroses.* In a psychosis the illness is obviously pathological and its manifestations are quite foreign to normal modes of thinking, feeling and behaving. In contrast, psychoneurotic symptoms often appear to be exaggerations or distortions of normal traits. With the onset of a psychosis there is usually a distinct break with the person's habitual mental state but in psychoneurosis the progression of the illness from the patient's normal personality is often readily discernible. Many psychotics lose touch with reality to a greater or lesser extent unless their illness is treated, whereas neurotics often (though not invariably) retain a good deal of uncomfortable insight into their condition. In general terms it can be said that the psychoses tend to be intense illnesses which are often associated with disturbed behaviour but the neuroses are less intense and are characterized more by the patient's internal suffering than by any marked abnormality of conduct.

Despite these broad differences between the two types of illness it must be admitted that their division into psychosis and neurosis is largely administrative and has little intrinsic meaning. There are so many exceptions to the criteria we have just mentioned for distinguishing them that the classification is almost useless. However, the terms are in common use in psychiatry and in the interests of communication we have to mention them. In some psychotic conditions (for example, many depressive illnesses) there is little or no disturbance of behaviour or thinking, the patient often retains good insight and he certainly suffers intensely. On the other hand, some psychoneurotics (such as severe hysterics) may be grossly histrionic in their behaviour, have a remarkable lack of insight and often make others suffer a good deal more than they do themselves. To complicate matters further, a proportion of neurotic disorders turn out to be due to underlying psychotic illnesses and one may merge into the other. In the course of your work you will undoubtedly use these terms, psychosis and neurosis. They are useful in helping to distinguish between broad types of illness, but you should not be persuaded that they are anything more than a convenient mnemonic.

General Features of the Psychoneuroses

It is important for social workers to know about psychoneurotic illnesses because, whatever their speciality, these are amongst the commonest conditions seen in the general population.

In Chapter 3 we discuss personality development and we point out that, in order to maintain its stability and its control over the primitive aspects of mental function, the ego has available a number of defence mechanisms. Any stress, however slight, will bring the defence system into action and the mature personality has a wide variety of responses which can be tailored to suit the situation. The unstable personality or the one which has been subjected to overwhelming stress will tend to rely too much on the small number of defences left available to it and if these defensive mechanisms are used repeatedly they may become habitual features of the personality. For example, one person may rely heavily on repression and unpleasant experiences are blotted from consciousness and apparently forgotten: another may employ the mechanism of projection and then all his failures are explained as being due to the malice of other people. If these are constantly in use in order to solve neurotic problems the whole personality may become tinged by their influence. If an individual is under stress there is a tendency for him to fall back on less and less mature forms of defence as the more sophisticated forms fail him. Thus an important facet of the psychoneurotic illness is this need to resort to immature or inappropriate modes of thought, emotion or behaviour at times of stress.

This regressive tendency is universal but if it is very marked it is usually the sign of unbalanced personality development. In some cases this is due to the individual's having been encouraged too much in one way and too little in another as when a child is expected to behave as a little adult long before his emotional equipment enables him to do so. In other people there may have been severe emotional traumata which have prevented an important part of the normal emotional development from occurring. In others again some form of inappropriate behaviour has been inadvertently encouraged: an otherwise normal child who has tantrums and whose parents invariably give in to these may grow up to face great difficulties because the continuance of the tantrums (or their equivalent) is viewed much less sympathetically by other people.

The neuroses are frequently associated with decreased efficiency in social functioning and disturbances in interpersonal relationships. Cause and effect are closely interwoven here. Possibly some difficulty in the person's early upbringing has produced an inability to be completely at ease in certain situations or with certain people. This may cause a certain amount of strain within the personality and render it more liable to breakdown. If a neurotic illness develops these disabilities increase and can lead to an almost complete interruption of personal and social relationships.

The concept of neurotic illness must always be a relative one. We all have neurotic traits but most of us can compensate for these or at least learn to avoid the anxiety-provoking situation: but everyone has a breaking point and this will be reached sooner or later if sufficient pressure is applied. Some people react neurotically to the slightest stress and others react only occasionally in this way, but the difference between these types of individual appears to be quantitative rather than qualitative. When the ego defences are put under strain the person becomes ill in that he is excessively tense and unhappy. But many people who feel like this do not

D

complain so their condition never comes to notice. Others complain more readily and their illness can be then recognized for what it is. The communication aspect of neurotic illness is important: the symptoms in themselves are a sort of distress signal but it is only if the patient complains that measures for treatment can be instituted.

We know from experience that when we have to face some difficulty we react with anxiety: this is normal and desirable because anxiety alerts us and makes us ready for action. But we know that some of the manifestations of anxiety, such as palpitations, muscular tension and diarrhoea, can be unpleasant. Usually these symptoms are related to a definite situation and disappear when the situation is resolved, but in some circumstances the anxiety may get out of control and may cause neurotic symptoms. Depending on the individual's predominant modes of defence the symptoms will appear as anxiety itself or as various other neurotic manifestations which are provoked by anxiety. There may be feelings of fear which at times reach panic level, and while the person knows these to be unreasonable emotions he has difficulty in controlling them. Not infrequently the fear is accompanied by an inexplicable feeling of impending disaster. If these symptoms become fixed they constitute a psychoneurotic illness. When this occurs the person is said to be in a state of *Psychic Conflict* and it is assumed that his ego defences have broken down in their struggle with the primitive demands of the id. This is a grossly oversimplified explanation of the genesis of neurotic illness, but we hope the account we have given provides an impression of how it arises and why it may take such different forms in various individuals.

We shall now consider the psychoneuroses under five main headings according to their main characteristics. The headings are Anxiety Neurosis, Neurotic Depression, Obsessional Neurosis, Phobic States and Hysteria. These conditions are not mutually exclusive and in many patients the symptoms are so mixed as to make diagnosis difficult, but it is important to make a diagnosis since each illness tends to have its own prospect for recovery and the treatment may vary according to the predominant symptoms.

Unfortunately, diagnosis is not based on objectively verifiable factors and it is often difficult to come to a definite conclusion in a particular case, but despite this the classification works fairly well in a rule-of-thumb kind of way.

1. *Anxiety Neurosis*

We have pointed out that anxiety is a natural and necessary reaction to stress. This stress may be external or it may occur within the individual's own mind. Sometimes it is acute, as when the person is placed in a dangerous situation (or what he perceives as danger—for example, moral danger) and he may react with panic which persists after the peril has passed. If this is severe and persists long enough to become habitual it is then an illness. Anxiety neurosis may also occur as the result of more prolonged pressures such as marital problems or other interpersonal difficulties, inability to cope with the responsibility of work, pressure of debt and so on. In these circumstances the onset is more gradual and the patient often suffers from a persistently grumbling type of anxiety with intermittent outbursts of acute panicky feelings. When no obvious precipitating factor is present it is likely that there is some kind of internal emotional conflict which is spilling over in the form of anxiety. In this type of case there is often evidence that the person has been habitually anxious and a chronic worrier: the illness is an exaggeration of these tendencies and grows out of them. Other personality features which seem to predispose to anxiety are an excessively rigid outlook and chronic irresolution in coming to decisions.

The patient with anxiety neurosis often presents with a multitude of complaints which may be predominantly psychic or physical. The psychic symptoms are particularly those of tension, fear, and apprehension. In addition the patient often feels restless and is unable to concentrate as well as usual. Despite the restlessness the incentive to tackle problems is reduced and there is undue apprehension about necessary decisions. Sleeplessness is common and he tosses and turns or else lies awake worrying about his problems. The appetite is often affected and the zest for food is lost. If the condition is not too severe the patient may be distracted from his worries for a time by company or diversions, but left to his own resources he soon begins to be anxious again. If the illness is prolonged he often becomes thoroughly disheartened and depressed and all the time there is an acute awareness of the symptoms, if not always of their cause.

The physical symptoms of anxiety neurosis are numerous and varied. Many of them are produced by excessive activity of the autonomic nervous system, that part of the nervous system through which the brain controls the internal functions of the body. The heart-rate speeds up and there may be palpitations; there may also be breathlessness and sometimes there is a feeling of discomfort or even pain in the chest. Loss of appetite, indigestion, nausea or even vomiting can occur and diarrhoea is common. The person often complains of headache, muscular pains and "pins and needles": giddiness and even fainting are sometimes present. The individual is often morbidly aware of all his bodily functions and is ready to complain at the slightest irregularity, including many quite normal phenomena that would usually pass unnoticed.

The diagnosis of anxiety neurosis always demands care because so many of the complaints are physical in nature that it is necessary to be sure that no organic disease is actually present. For example, thyrotoxicosis (overactivity of the thyroid gland) can produce almost exactly similar symptoms and it may be necessary to perform biochemical investigations to exclude its presence: other debilitating illnesses can also produce similar effects. Apart from physical illness, anxiety occurs as a symptom in a number of psychiatric conditions and these must always be looked for: they include depressive illness, schizophrenia, obsessional neurosis and the early stages of dementing illnesses. Obviously the treatment of the anxiety symptoms becomes of secondary importance when another condition is present and the anxiety will usually disappear when the other illness is cured.

The course of the illness is variable. Some acute forms last only a few days while others may go on for many years. The acute form may require no treatment other than tactful handling if it has been the result of a single episode of severe emotional trauma, but if the symptoms seem to be persisting some form of abreaction therapy is often very successful. With this type of treatment the patient is induced to a state of near-sleep by means of relaxation, drugs or hypnosis. Then when the excessively alerted ego defences have been lulled the person is encouraged to re-experience the traumatic event with its attendant emotions. In the safety of the therapeutic situation he may be able to discharge all the fears attached to the trauma and thus make a complete recovery, but the method usually only works if it is carried out within a comparatively short time. In the more chronic forms of anxiety any aggravating factors should be dealt with. If physical or other psychiatric illnesses are present they should be treated and practical help should be given with any environmental difficulties which are perpetuating the symptoms. In particular the individual should be encouraged and helped to make necessary decisions instead of repeatedly shelving them. He must be prevented from becoming a chronically hypochondriacal invalid. Tranquillizers often give a good deal of symptomatic relief and night-sedation will improve the sleep. Often there is a need for psychotherapy which in simpler cases may be purely supportive but which may need to be interpretative in cases where there is considerable emotional conflict. When interpersonal difficulties are prominent, group psychotherapy may be indicated. Throughout treatment the patient needs a great deal of moral support until anxiety is sufficiently under control to enable him to function normally once more.

2. *Neurotic Depression*

In Chapter 9 we describe the type of depressive illness which occurs in manic-depressive psychosis. In that condition the depression of mood is often extremely severe and is associated with symptoms such as retardation, guilt feelings, suicidal tendencies and, at times, delusions. These features warrant the illness being included amongst the functional psychoses.

However, depression does not necessarily constitute an illness. Variations in mood-state are part of normal experience and it is normal to be dejected when one has been particularly disappointed or reprimanded, just as it is normal to be jubilant on receiving a piece of particularly good news. Internal events can also strongly influence one's frame of mind and we all know how depressing a persistent worry or a persistent pain can be: that unaccountable "Monday morning blues" feeling is a common experience, as is a period of gloom following a physical illness like influenza. Usually mood swings of this sort are short-lived and do not interfere with one's normal mental processes or with one's social behaviour, but there are occasions when a more severe stress or a more prolonged worry may precipitate a rather more marked mood change, perhaps lasting for several days. Grief after a bereavement usually involves feelings of depression: here the depression is part of the process the person undergoes when the emotions which were invested in the deceased individual begin to be detached. In the bereavement situation the depression usually lifts fairly soon if the person is allowed to work through the grief process and is allowed to express the sense of loss. This sort of depressive reaction is understandable and should not usually be regarded as an illness. It usually disappears of its own accord and it requires sympathetic handling rather than treatment in most cases.

Some depressive reactions do not resolve so quickly, either because the cause of the depression remains or because the individual does not have sufficient resources of personality with which to combat it. Sometimes the causative factor is relatively slight and then it has to be assumed that the person has some predisposition to depression in his personality make-up. When the depressive symptoms persist like this they may be sufficiently obvious to be regarded as an illness, which is often referred to as a reactive depression. This type of illness is seen much more by general practitioners than by psychiatrists because it is rarely severe enough to necessitate the patient's attending hospital. The mood is not usually very depressed and it often responds favourably to environmental stimuli, though there is a tendency for the person to relapse into a state of dejection afterwards. The patient finds that when he is alone he is apt to brood and feel miserable but if he is engaged in some activity or mixing in company there is a marked rise in his spirits for the time being. He is rarely retarded in thought or action and indeed it is quite common for the depression to be accompanied by anxiety, agitation and overactivity, though these symptoms may also fluctuate in their severity. Appetite may or may not be affected but sleep is often restless and disturbed. Although the depression is usually not very profound, suicidal thoughts are sometimes present and some patients do make suicidal attempts. These attempts may be quite serious and it is never wise to neglect threats of suicide.

The outlook in reactive depression usually depends on how soon the precipitating factor disappears or is dealt with. In the case of an external stress, alteration of the patient's social environment may be the key factor, but when the stress is due to emotional conflicts some form of psychotherapy is often necessary to resolve these.

In some patients the form of not-too-severe depression we have been describing occurs in association with prominent psycho-neurotic symptoms like anxiety, phobic fears or hysterical phenomena. These neurotic features may be quite foreign to the individual's normal personality, but in some cases they indicate the presence of an habitually unstable personality whose characteristics are thrown into relief by the presence of depression. Where neurotic features are prominent the illness may be called *Neurotic Depression*, but this is an unsatisfactory diagnostic category because it may include a thoroughly mixed group of illnesses whose only common factor is the presence of some degree of depression.

Apart from the possibility of suicidal attempts, the relatively mild but persistent depression should never be neglected because it is sometimes the prelude to a more serious psychotic depressive illness. It is rarely possible to predict which patient with reactive depression will ultimately develop a severer condition, but those people who have a previous history of manic-depressive psychosis or a family history of such an illness should be carefully observed. It is difficult to prove, but it is tempting to think that one could forestall the onset of severe manic-depressive illness by applying antidepressant treatment in such cases while their disorder is still relatively mild.

In mild cases of neurotic depression, reassurance and support are all that are required and if the patient's morale is prevented from slumping the condition will eventually tend to improve spontaneously. As always, help with environmental problems may be important, but as much as possible the patient should be encouraged to solve these by his own efforts. Psychotherapy may be needed, often to deal with the neurotic problems as much as the depression. Antidepressant drugs, which are often very valuable in treating severe depression, are relatively ineffective in these milder depressive conditions largely because they do not treat the neurotic part of the symptomatology, but partly because, in themselves, they cannot solve nagging problems. Some neurotic depressives tend to become chronic regardless of the treatment given. Their illness is rarely completely incapacitating, but they tend to lead unhappy, frustrating lives, often driving relatives and friends into an equally miserable state by their constant irritability and complaining. Some of them become incorrigible hypochondriacs, forever pestering their doctors for treatments but never gaining any relief of symptoms. Many of these individuals are inadequate people at the best of times and their illness is perhaps a way of getting support and reassurance which unfortunately never satisfies them. It takes great patience to deal with this type of situation, but a friendly and capable social worker can often keep such patients reasonably well by means of judicious encouragement. Support like this is sometimes sufficient to prevent periodic relapses which would otherwise result in admission to hospital.

3. *Obsessional Neurosis*

This condition is also known as obsessive-compulsive disorder and its main characteristics are obsessional thoughts or impulses which the individual knows are irrational and which he tries to dispel. Insight is not affected and while the ideas often seem inappropriate to the personality they do not have the bizarre quality which is present in delusion. Nevertheless, they constantly intrude on consciousness and the patient cannot rid himself of them no matter how hard he resists their presence.

We all experience obsessional symptoms in mild form at some time or another: it is quite common to find a snatch of tune running through one's head again and again till it becomes quite maddening or to be unable to stop doing a jig-saw puzzle until one has put the last piece in place even though there are more important things to do. At worst these forms of behaviour are a nuisance and they do not interfere seriously with one's normal life. Most of these mild compulsions are regarded as normal and are fairly harmless. Children often go through a stage of development when compulsive rituals are very prominent: these may consist of avoiding the lines on the pavement, repeating certain phrases several times in a fixed order, touching railings or a variety of other behaviours. All of this seems to be associated with a preoccupation with orderliness which is a normal phase in the child's psychic development and an important mechanism in enabling him to control his environment. Presumably it also helps to lay down the basis for the type of persistent behaviour which adults require in order to form lasting emotional attachments and pursue long-term plans.

None of us completely abandons this obsessional stage of development, but some people are especially prone to grow up with marked compulsive traits, perhaps because an emotional trauma has caused a fixation of libido at this particular level or perhaps because over-conscientious parents have laid undue stress on the development of habits such as orderliness, cleanliness. regular bowel habit, self-denial and punctiliousness. The result may be a person with distinctly obsessional traits in his personality but no illness or someone whose compulsions eventually take command and result in an obsessional neurosis. Commonly, but not invariably, this form of illness arises in individuals who already have a decidedly obsessional type of personality.

According to psychoanalytic theory the obsessional possesses an over-strong and unyielding superego which produces a severely moral attitude. When an obsessional neurosis develops it re-awakens unresolved emotional conflicts which have occurred at the anal-sadistic stage of libidinal development and this produces a release of primitive aggression which is unacceptable to the ego and superego. An unconscious attempt is made to displace this emotion on to some more acceptable situation and as a result the person may become fanatically opposed to immorality or may develop a pathological fear of contamination by dirt or disease. Unworthy thoughts and actions are denied by "undoing" rituals which often have symbolic significance, as when the obsessional repeatedly washes in order to avoid all forms of physical or psychological uncleanliness. Unfortunately the rituals rarely dispel the fears completely and in an attempt to bring them under control these ritualized actions become more pervasive and demanding: whereas it was once possible to be clean for a while by washing three times in succession, it may now need to be three times three and so on until the person's whole life is spent scrubbing himself unavailingly. This type of individual is engaged in the hopeless task of being perfectly good because he cannot tolerate a normal amount of aggression or sexual emotion. Some patients go to the extreme of becoming quite immobile and even their simplest action becomes endlessly prolonged because of its implications which need to be minutely considered.

Obsessional phenomena may be limited to the area of intellect and emotion and may take the form of persistent mental rumination on some topic, a compulsion to count or tabulate, or a constant doubting of the person's own capabilities. There is often a great deal of preoccupation with health matters and, in particular, with bowel function: a great deal of anxiety may arise if there is the mildest degree of constipation or diarrhoea and the obsessional will expatiate lyrically on the regularity or irregularity with which his bowel performs. Sometimes, as well as obsessional thoughts there may be compulsive deeds. As already noted, excessive washing may occur or the individual may have to check and re-check his work for possible mistakes. Sometimes the patient becomes aware of severe aggressive urges towards certain people and he becomes very afraid that he might be compelled to harm them. It is not common for the obsessional to give way to such impulses, but occasionally the illness does take antisocial forms: for example, the patient may steal compulsively, and quite often this is done in a conspicuous way as though he were inviting punishment. Presumably this represents a child-like belief that severe retribution will atone for his unworthy thoughts.

(The relationship of obsessional rituals to magical and religious ceremonials has often been discussed. It has been pointed out that they all contain an underlying element of the wish to ward off possible evil or disaster by taking part in carefully designed propitiation rites: unless these rites are absolutely correct their mystical effectiveness is lost, which seems to represent the child's desire to create order out of chaos. However, we should point out here that religious ritual and religion are not necessarily synonymous, and the great majority of people who participate in either are certainly not suffering from obsessional neurosis.)

While obsessional neurosis does sometimes arise in a person whose previous personality has displayed little in the way of compulsive features, it is true to say that the illness is quite often an exacerbation of long-standing traits. Obsessional personalities are common in the general population and such people are valuable on account of their thriftiness, punctuality and sense of responsibility. But sometimes these habits are carried to extremes and then the individual tends to be rigid, unyielding and over-perfectionistic. His judgements are harsh and he is intolerant of any hint of sensuality. His life runs to an unalterable pattern and he may have set routines to which he invariably closely adheres. In some cases, he is a collector or a hoarder. In psychoanalytic terms he is known as an "Anal Personality" and in German psychiatry he is described as an "Anankastic Personality", but both these terms are in effect synonymous with the phrase "Obsessional Personality" which is most widely used. Such a person is not ill, but if his demands on himself become too severe he may begin to break down into an obsessional neurosis. Then there is a marked increase in tension and the ritualistic defences become progressively more pervasive and disabling.

There is possibly an hereditary element in obsessional neurosis. Certainly, obsessional characteristics often run in families and sometimes there are cases of the illness in different generations of the same family. However, it is uncertain how much of this is due to constitutional factors and how much is due to prevailing attitudes within a household. It is probable that an over-strict upbringing can lay the foundations of the condition by placing too much emphasis on self-control. In many cases the obsessional's training has taught him to be inflexible and to view things in uncompromising black and white terms.

Obsessional neurosis usually comes on gradually and the sufferer, being obsessional, almost invariably fights the symptoms till they become totally uncontrollable. Only when he has broken down does he seek help. At this stage the patient is likely to be in his twenties or early thirties, but his illness has probably been present for many years already. Sometimes the actual breakdown is almost fortuitous, perhaps brought about by a bereavement or a physical illness: in these cases what appears to be a precipitating factor may only be the means by which the condition has been revealed. The illness causes an enormous amount of distress to the patient and the compulsive symptoms are so unremitting that life becomes totally bound down and circumscribed. Each day is a grey and dismal round of unrelenting rituals whose presence causes tension and the resistance to which intensifies the tension. The course of the neurosis differs in various people: it may become progressively worse till it completely disables the sufferer or it may fluctuate in its severity. Some cases have an alternation of marked obsessionalism with periods of normality and when this occurs one should always suspect the possibility that it is actually a disguised form of depression. Occasionally the compulsive symptoms begin to develop a bizarre quality and in such cases there is a strong possibility that there is an incipient schizophrenia underlying the neurosis.

Most of the mild cases of obsessional neurosis probably clear up in time, but the outlook in severe cases tends to be rather poor. A proportion of patients do certainly recover, but often this really means that the compulsions remain and the patient learns to live with them without too much tension. When the person comes to medical attention he is often depressed, having been worn down by the pressure of symptoms. If this is so, antidepressant treatment with drugs or electroconvulsive therapy (see p. 213) may produce some degree of relief. It is always important to take an optimistic attitude with the patient because any improvement in his morale will help him to cope that much better with his problems. Because of the obsessional's staying power suicide is uncommon, but eventually some people do succumb to the illness and kill themselves.

Treatment is largely designed to enable the individual to overcome the effect of the obsessions, and is mostly supportive in nature. One should always provide encouragement and help with any environmental problems which are complicating the situation. Drugs can be very useful in reducing tension and treating depression, but psychotherapy is usually relatively unsuccessful because the patient inevitably denies his conflicts and this interferes with insight. In a small number of grossly disabled cases pre-frontal leucotomy may need to be carried out: this operation consists of removal of a portion of the frontal region of the brain in order to destroy certain inhibiting and tension-producing mechanisms. Because of the ethical and practical problems attached to such a procedure it is only carried out if no other therapy is practicable.

It is not easy to generalize about the type of social work required in dealing with obsessional neurosis. Certainly the worker requires a positive and understanding approach towards the patient. The obsessional often tries to be independent and may politely reject help, but when the illness has become severe he may be unable to work and he and his family may need a great deal of aid. Fortunately he usually strives as hard as he can to regain his independence, but during the course of the illness various practical problems may arise: for example, a mother may be filled with such a degree of self-doubt that she cannot take the responsibility of tending her infant; a housewife may be so afraid of contamination by dirt that she cannot go out to do her shopping; or a woman may be so methodical about household tasks that she spends all day tackling the first chore and nothing else gets done. In situations like these the patient suffers intensely and a social worker's practical help and encouragement can be of great value in supporting the obsessional through the bleak periods when life seems insupportable.

93

4. *Phobic States*

A phobia is an unreasonable fear associated with some situation, object or idea. The fear tends to recur each time the person encounters the situation (or even thinks about it) and in severe cases can give rise to attacks of panic. The patient is well aware that the fear is irrational, but is quite unable to control it.

Mild phobic symptoms regularly crop up in everyday life and we do not think it particularly abnormal if a person is afraid of insects, the dark, heights, enclosed spaces and so on. Usually these fears are relatively slight and either it is possible to control them or else the situation which causes them can be avoided without inconvenience. In some people the fear is a good deal more acute than this or it is difficult for them to avoid the anxiety-provoking circumstances: for example, if a man earns his living by being a steeplejack and for some reason becomes afraid of heights he will be forced each day to face something which terrifies him. In this case, the intense fear is focused on one situation and the person may be perfectly normal otherwise. In other patients the fear is much more generalized and these people become panicky in a whole variety of circumstances. Obviously this latter type of phobic disturbance is very disabling because there is always likely to be something in the environment causing fear.

The phobia may be regarded as a special form of obsessional symptom in which a negative compulsion is operating to force the patient to avoid some situation, but phobic illnesses and obsessional illnesses are quite dissimilar in many ways. Phobias appear to arise in several ways. Certain fears are natural in children and serve a useful function: avoidance of wriggling, snake-like objects is a normal reaction in a toddler and in rural societies where snakes may be encountered such a mode of behaviour could have a definite life-preserving function. Sometimes this sort of fear fails to resolve as it should and the adult may be left with an unreasonable loathing of "creepie-crawlies". In other people, aversion to a situation has been produced by some traumatic event: near-drowning may cause a fear of entering the water, or being locked in a small room as a punishment may later cause panic in enclosed spaces. At times the phobia appears to have a symbolic function and may disguise another fear which for some reason is unacceptable to the ego. An example of this last type is the case of the woman who becomes afraid to leave her house because of forbidden sexual desires within herself: unconsciously she equates going into the street with going on to the street and the street becomes a place where these dangerous desires might gain expression; so it is safer to remain at home. In the case of some children who refuse to go to school it is less because they are afraid of school and more because they are terrified that when they are away from home some catastrophe will happen to their parents. Some patients may develop acute fears of knives and other weapons and it is only on investigation that it becomes obvious that they have extremely aggressive feelings towards someone and feel very guilty about this: in their ambivalence they wish the other person harm, but are afraid that something unpleasant might really happen so they shun any thought of violence and become afraid of instruments of violence.

Phobic illness often arises in someone who has had more than her fair share of mild phobic fears previously and the condition may develop gradually from one of these fears or may suddenly develop after some frightening incident. Sometimes the fear develops as part of an obsessional illness as when a person fears contamination by dirt and takes elaborate steps to avoid being soiled. This may involve the avoidance of certain places or activities and if it is not possible to do this there may be acute feelings of panic. In whatever way the phobia arises it tends to be perpetuated by psychological stresses and to be improved by removal of the stress, but there are occasions when it becomes self-perpetuating and relatively independent of external circumstances. The patient is often ashamed of his unreasonable fears and tries to hide them till this is no longer possible. Very often a great deal of diffuse anxiety accompanies the illness and some patients develop quite severe feelings of depression and *Depersonalization*. (This last is an unpleasant feeling of detachment from one's surroundings and of unreality.) If depersonalization is present and is severe it is usually a rather ominous sign and the illness tends to be slower in clearing up.

The treatment of phobic illnesses usually begins with the giving of sedation and reassurance and this may be enough to effect cure in many milder cases. Often, some form of psychotherapy is required and, particularly in intelligent patients, analysis of their basic difficulties can be very successful in bringing about improvement. In less intelligent patients with reduced capacity for insight, direct suggestion and hypnosis may be valuable. In all cases, environmental stress factors should be remedied where possible since a reduction in general tension usually causes some relief of the phobic fears. Nowadays, various forms of conditioning therapy (see p. 107) are becoming more widely used in the treatment of phobias, especially in that type of phobia where the fear is restricted to a specific situation. An attempt is made to "desensitize" the individual psychologically by teaching him progessively to relax in the presence of the stress-factor and in successful cases the individual becomes quite free of the particular anxiety. When the fear is more widespread and diffuse it is often a good deal more difficult to define and treat it in this way. Behaviour therapy is a purely symptomatic form of treatment and makes little attempt to deal with causative factors, but despite this its protagonists claim very striking results for it in the treatment of some phobic conditions and this is certainly borne out in our experience.

5. *Hysteria*

This illness is usually given great prominence in psychiatric textbooks, but severe hysteria is not a common illness and nowadays seems to be becoming even less common. It is interesting to psychiatrists because its manifestations are often dramatic and the illness inhabits a kind of no-man's land between psychiatry and neurology, between mind and body. Hysteria is a psychoneurotic condition in which a wide variety of psychological symptoms occur and in which there may be prominent physical signs and symptoms in the absence of a demonstrable organic illness. There is a marked tendency to utilize the psychological mechanisms of regression, dissociation and conversion and at an unconscious level the illness is employed to effect some kind of gain (see below). In the layman's mind hysteria is synonymous with disturbed and noisy behaviour, and while this does occur it is only one facet of the condition. As used by many people hysteria is a term of abuse, but as we use it, it describes a particular form of disorder.

In hysterical illness there is much regression to immature forms of behaviour and there may be sulkiness, petulance, tantrums and other forms of attention-seeking. Very often this is unconsciously designed to enable the patient to gain some end and to manipulate other people into giving her attention. This is very like a child's behaviour and it is also the sort of thing which may be found in someone who is physically unwell or excessively tired and also in old people who are becoming a little childish. Hysteria is seen more often in women than in men. It has often been remarked that immature behaviour and emotion tend to go with immature physique: it is certainly striking how often fragile little doll-like people have fragile doll-like emotions.

At times the patient's behaviour is quite the opposite from attention-seeking and instead she is unnaturally calm and undisturbed, at least on the surface. In this state the emotional conflict is still raging underneath, but for the time being it has been possible to repress and deny it. The calmness, which is known as "la Belle Indifférence", is extremely fragile and easily shattered, but sometimes it can deceive one into thinking that the patient is really enjoying a period of tranquillity. In severe hysteria the denial may go even further and in some cases the individual develops amnesia and can wander off, apparently unaware of her surroundings. This is not a permanent loss of memory, but is rather a repression of some unpalatable truth: the attempt to deny it is so thoroughgoing that for the time being *everything* is repressed. Sometimes hysterical symptoms can be so bizarre that they may be mistaken for other mental illnesses, and they may even mimic dementia on occasions. In other instances the patient may complain of physical symptoms and develop quite dramatic signs. Some patients develop paralyses, skin rashes, pseudo-epileptic seizures, anaesthetic areas of skin which are temporarily insusceptible to painful stimuli, or even pseudo-pregnancies. These "Conversion Symptoms" can sometimes be very convincing and the patient herself is certainly convinced about them while they last. It is important that the medical practitioner should not be misled into ignoring their psychological basis.

Under sufficient stress an hysterical illness can arise in a previously normal individual, but quite frequently it is an exacerbation of the features of a pre-existing hysterical personality (see p. 126) and when this is so the precipitating factors may be relatively slight. A slight thwarting of the patient's wishes or a mild environmental difficulty may be enough to produce histrionic complaints, attention-demanding behaviour and numerous other complaints quite out of proportion to the reality of the situation. When someone is as ready as this to rush into psychiatric illness it is likely that other people will eventually become tired of her and the effectiveness of her symptoms as a means of summoning help usually diminishes with time. Then the complaints become more flamboyant and suicidal threats and gestures may be made. These may not be seriously intended but, by accident or otherwise, a small proportion succeed so it is never safe to ignore a threat of suicide: at the same time it is important not to give in to the patient's moral blackmail if this is at all possible.

Hysteria may be due predominantly to constitutional or to psychological causes. In the former category are those patients with markedly immature physique, immature brain-wave patterns as measured by the electroencephalogram or a strong family history of neurotic illness. In the psychologically precipitated group, psychoanalytic theory postulates that fixation of libido has occurred at the genital stage of emotional development and that under stress there will be a resurgence of Oedipal conflicts. Incestuous desires are re-awakened which are intolerable to the ego and they have to be repressed. In this process the conflicts are dissociated and converted to other psychological complaints or physical symptoms. This diversion of psychic tension produces immediate relief from anxiety which is the *Primary Gain* of the illness. If the illness receives attention from other people this may give a kind of satisfaction to the patient and in these circumstances the symptoms may become prolonged in order to obtain this type of *Secondary Gain*. Sometimes the differentiation between this process and malingering is exceedingly tenuous and this perpetuation of complaints is commonly seen in cases where there is prolonged litigation for accident compensation. However, in true hysteria the mechanisms are mostly unconscious and the tension symptoms are not feigned.

There seems little doubt that a disturbed upbringing often contributes to the predisposition towards hysterical illness. The emotionally deprived child or the child who has suffered repeated emotional traumata in infancy appears particularly liable to develop the condition subsequently. The tendency may remain hidden and may be evoked by a natural event such as the increase in the force of the sexual emotions at the time of puberty or by a relatively fortuitous occurrence in adult life such as emotional or physical trauma or debilitating physical illness. Sometimes the precipitating factor is the onset of another psychiatric illness such as depression or schizophrenia and when the diagnosis of hysteria is being made it is always necessary to consider the possibility of their underlying presence.

If the basic personality is neurotic, hysterical symptoms may become chronic, especially if the secondary gain is particularly satisfying to the individual, as when she has become a pampered invalid. The treatment of hysteria is usually most satisfactory when an underlying cause can be dealt with, whether it be a stress situation, a physical disorder or another mental illness. Psychotherapy may be employed in treatment, but it is frequently unsuccessful because of the patient's lack of insight and propensity for denial, and, in general, the lower the intelligence the poorer the effect of this treatment. Physical treatments are usually to be avoided since their effect in hysteria is often simply to cause side-effects which provide the basis for further physical complaints, but tranquillizing drugs are useful in reducing the level of anxiety. The patient's suggestibility would make one think that hypnosis could be a useful form of therapy, but its results are frequently transitory and the wholesale removal of symptoms (which are a form of psychic defence) may have adverse effects if the anxiety seeks other channels of expression. Abreactive techniques (see p. 108) are sometimes successful when the illness has been caused by an acute traumatic experience.

Since many hysterics are immature and socially inept they may need a great deal of support in their problems. Like children, they always try to take the easy way out of a situation, but help should be directed towards enabling them to solve their own problems. The social worker should not be manipulated into making the patient's decisions, though with the best will in the world she will find it impossible to avoid this all the time. The hysteric usually exaggerates difficulties and it must be made clear to her that any help that is given will be on a realistic level: never be persuaded to make impracticable promises and do not succumb to the patient's various forms of emotional blackmail. The approach should mainly be a judicious mixture of kindness and firmness. Hysterics are often difficult and trying people and in the more chronic cases work with them may be relatively unrewarding. Nevertheless, a consistent and continuing approach to their troubles may well avert numerous crises and consequent nervous breakdowns.

Treatment of the Psychoneuroses

Most cases of psychoneurosis never need to attend a psychiatrist. The mildest forms quickly clear up of their own accord, but when a patient does need to seek medical help he will most likely receive this from his own doctor. Usually it is only the most serious cases of neurosis or the individuals who complain most persistently who are referred to the psychiatrist by the general practitioner. Even nowadays, a great many miserable people do not realize that their unhappiness is due to an emotional illness and they never seek the help of a doctor: they either suffer in silence, dose themselves with patent medicines or repeatedly seek reassurance from friends or acquaintances. In the course of your professional and private lives you are bound to find people coming to you because they know that you are a social worker, asking for advice and help in their problems. When this happens it is important to distinguish the problem from the person's reaction to it. Is the problem a real one, is it as serious as the individual makes out, is it of his own making or not? Often his anxiety can be put to rest by reassurance or by some simple piece of practical intervention. When this is so, you should be at some pains to let him know that you do not regard him as a client but rather that you are offering help purely on a good-neighbour basis. Otherwise, if you take his anxieties too seriously, you may persuade him that he is ill when he is not and you yourself will be in danger of having him become over-dependent on you.

Conversely it is just as important not to miss a severe neurotic reaction which is perhaps overshadowed by the apparent magnitude of some problem. It is common for patients to express their anxiety by asking for advice on some difficulty, but this is really an excuse to enable them to communicate their distress to someone they think may help them. Advice and practical help should never be withheld where it is needed, but gratuitous and inappropriate advice is always to be avoided. It is tempting to tell an unhappy woman that what she needs is another child, an anxious man that he should change to less responsible work, or a vacillating individual that it is time he "picked himself up" and started to make his own decisions. If the failure of these people to cope is due to psychiatric illness they will get nothing but dissatisfaction from trying to follow misguided advice. Many psychoneurotic patients report that they have been trying to follow the exhortations of friends and relatives for a long time before seeking psychiatric advice and their inability to succeed has only intensified their guilt and agitation. The experienced social worker usually knows which needs the more attention, the patient or his problem, but it is always worth emphasizing the potential dangers of seeing illness where it does not exist or, on the other hand, offering a sick individual an ineffective substitute for treatment.

Psychology and psychiatry are subjects of great inherent interest and it is fascinating to probe the minds and motives of other people, whether they are acquaintances, patients or even professional colleagues. Insight into the motives of oneself or of others can be of great value in psychiatry and social work, but it is possible to carry this enquiry to excessive lengths. Our aim is to help the client or patient as humanely and as efficiently as possible, and ultimately our suitability for our work will depend less on the details of our own motivations and personality traits and more on whether we can get ahead with the task in hand and complete it to the patient's and our own satisfaction. Too much introspection can paralyse a social worker's initiative and can seriously interfere with her efficiency in her field. She has to make decisions and she has to maintain friendly contact and regular communication with medical and other colleagues. She can only do this properly by having confidence in herself and in the usefulness of her work. Her practical contribution should complement and support whatever treatment the patient is receiving and to be effective the social worker should understand the significance of the various forms of therapy. Let us now consider these in turn.

Supportive Treatment

In cases where the patient is suffering from a psychoneurotic illness, but is not severely disabled by it, the simplest form of treatment may be the most appropriate and this need not necessarily be carried through by a psychiatrist. Reassurance, lending a sympathetic ear, being readily available at a time of crisis, not moralizing or condemning, are all valuable services which the social worker can provide. Many patients gain huge relief from tension just by being able to pour out their troubles to someone who really understands. When a patient's difficulties are long-continuing and he is chronically unable to cope, the social worker may be a psychological crutch whose presence can restore confidence and provide a stable point of reference. But even in the most inadequate individuals the aim should be to develop their self-reliance so that ultimately they will learn to be independent.

The Psychotherapies

In the course of psychotherapy the patient is encouraged to talk out his problems and to express the emotions which are associated with them. By letting him do this the therapist believes that repressed feelings which have been causing tension and ill-health can be released and that, by gaining insight into these, the patient can adapt better to life and its problems. Psychoneurotic illness is seen as an interference with the normal process of personality maturation and intervention by psychotherapy allows this process to be resumed.

Psychoanalysis. The treatment derived from the psychological theories of Sigmund Freud is the parent of most of the innumerable forms of psychotherapy. It is conducted by a psychoanalyst who is usually a psychiatrist (though some laymen may be allowed to qualify) and who has himself undergone a personal course of psychoanalysis as part of his long training. The patient is encouraged to *Free Associate*, that is, to relax and to speak out the thoughts which filter into consciousness on the principle that troublesome thoughts and emotions will emerge and be recognized for what they are in the security of the consulting rooms. To facilitate this process the patient is placed in a kind of sensory vacuum: the treatment is carried out in a quiet room, often with subdued light, and the patient is allowed to say what he wishes without inhibition. The psychoanalyst remains out of sight so that his physical presence will not interfere with the flow of the patient's fantasies. He intervenes as little as possible and then only to explain and interpret the material produced by the patient. The treatment encourages an *Emotional Catharsis*, the release and expression of long-repressed feelings, in order that the individual's emotional systems will re-align themselves in a more mature fashion. The patient re-enacts his interpersonal difficulties by developing fantasied relationships with the therapist so that at one time there may be a love, at another time a hate, attitude towards him. The therapist analyses this *Transference Situation* with the patient and uses it to explain to him that many of his difficulties are due to warped attitudes produced by earlier emotional difficulties. If the patient is able to gain insight he may then be able to adjust his attitudes to obtain satisfaction in real-life situations.

Psychoanalysis is a prolonged and time-consuming process which by its nature is restricted to a small number of cases. In order to obtain a full course of treatment the individual may be required to spend up to 5 hours a week for 3 or more years. He must also be prepared to stand the high financial cost of the therapy except in the relatively rare instances where free health service or charity treatment is available, so this means that it is mostly available to those in the higher socio-economic bracket. There are other restrictions on the receiving of psychoanalysis: the patient must be reasonably intelligent and must be able to verbalize his thoughts fluently, he must be strongly motivated to pursue such a prolonged process, and he must be suffering from one of the small number of psychoneurotic conditions which is susceptible to the treatment. If his basic personality is too unstable he is unlikely to be accepted for treatment because this is regarded as a bad prognostic sign: Freud himself regarded the most suitable case as being a person with a reasonable degree of education and a fairly reliable character.

Psychoanalytic teachings have had an enormous influence on western civilization: it is still widely debated as to whether the effect has been on balance good. Aside from purely social consequences, Freud's original work highlighted the hitherto largely ignored field of psychoneurotic illness and for many years psychoanalysis seemed to hold out hope for the rational treatment of many psychiatric illnesses by psychological means. Except among some enthusiasts much of this hope has faded and, as we have indicated above, most psychiatrists now regard its effective use as being restricted to a fairly narrow spectrum of neurotic conditions and personality disorders. It has never been possible to obtain scientific proof of the treatment's efficacy and it is admitted, even by its practitioners, that it is very difficult to be sure that the patient will ultimately benefit from it even when all the indications appear right. In fact, some psychoanalysts now say that their methods are not really a form of treatment for illness, but rather a means of gaining maturity, insight and self-fulfilment.

Other forms of psychotherapy. Since few people can undergo psychoanalysis and comparatively few of these can be expected to receive benefits from it commensurate with the trouble it involves, numerous attempts have been made to devise shorter and more effective forms of the treatment. These are given the general title of psychotherapy to distinguish them from classical psychoanalysis but the basic assumptions are usually derived from the teachings of Freud and his pupils (both faithful and apostate). The techniques vary widely with each form but most psychotherapies are described as "directive" forms of treatment because the therapist intervenes much more frequently and offers more directive advice and interpretation. He guides the patient's associations in what he regards as the appropriate direction and he facilitates this process by encouragement, exhortation and even aggressiveness. Most psychiatrists conduct some form of psychotherapy in their practices, sometimes adhering to a particular theoretical school, but more often nowadays using whatever approach seems most appropriate for the individual patient. Drugs, relaxation techniques and direct suggestion are frequently used in conjunction with psychotherapy if they are required. There is really no room in modern psychiatry for the theoretical purist who refuses to employ more than one treatment: psychiatric illness is too distressing for the patient to be allowed to continue with his symptoms longer than necessary and there are far too many individuals needing help for the psychiatrist to indulge his academic fancies at their expense.

Giving help and support to a patient constitutes a form of psychotherapy which the social worker is continually engaged in. For this reason she needs to have a well-balanced personality, an ability to empathize with other people and an adequate insight into her relationships with clients and colleagues. She should certainly not have a quasi-religious faith in the magic healing properties of any particular treatment or a tendency to become too embroiled in the psychodynamics of her case-work. She should appreciate that psychiatry has already passed through the painful and traumatic process of learning that it cannot place all its therapeutic eggs in one basket!

Group therapy. This form of psychotherapy is conducted with a number of patients at a time (usually up to ten but more in some circumstances). The obvious advantage is that it is much more economical of the therapist's time and allows him to deal with many more patients, but there are many individuals who cannot accept the group situation or whose illnesses are not suitable for this type of treatment. The technique is especially valuable for patients who have to be helped to function better in a social setting, who have to become less egocentric or who could gain insight into their own problems by sharing in the problems of others. Some groups are suitable for the employment of interpretative methods whereas others are more for a fairly superficial airing and discussion of mutual problems. Group therapy is used a good deal in the treatment of minor neuroses such as phobic illnesses and also in personality disorders. As well as this it can be very useful in helping some excessively shy and withdrawn patients to socialize, no matter what their diagnosis may be.

The therapeutic environment. In this concept the hospital or clinic, the staff and the patients themselves are all regarded as therapeutic agents. The aim of treatment is to encourage recovery by helping the patient to develop his social potential, to take responsibilities and to help others. A great deal of activity is conducted on informal and formal group therapy lines: the patient is kept very much in contact with other human beings and every attempt is made to prevent his becoming institutionalized. There is no doubt that in doing this the therapeutic community concept can be a valuable adjunct to specific treatment. Some people would go further and say that it is a form of therapy in its own right but we ourselves do not feel that this claim is fully justified.

Drug Treatment in the Psychoneuroses

Nowadays various types of drugs play an important part in the treatment of psychoneuroses and the fact that we mention them briefly is simply because the social worker is not directly concerned with their use. One of the most important groups consists of the various forms of tranquillizers which can reduce anxiety without producing undue drowsiness. Sedative drugs* to calm the patient and promote sleep are also used a great deal (and in fact used to

---

* In medical parlance sleeping drugs are often called hypnotics (this term refers to their sleep-inducing properties and has nothing to do with hypnosis).

excess by too many people). Antidepressant drugs are used mostly in severe depression but can be valuable in some cases of neurotic depression and obsessional neurosis. All of these substances produce mainly symptomatic relief, but this is often all that is required and in cases where other forms of treatment such as psychotherapy are also needed the drugs can make life more tolerable until recovery begins to take place. Patients are notoriously unreliable with drugs, either persistently forgetting to take them or sometimes taking more than the prescribed dose. A social worker should learn to recognize when the patient is neglecting or abusing his drugs and if she suspects this is happening she should encourage the patient to return to the proper regime and she should inform the doctor of what is happening.

(There is a group of stimulant drugs which can be used to provide a temporary increase in energy and also to help in weight reduction—because they inhibit the appetite. These have been employed in the past for the treatment of various neurotic conditions, but there is no longer any indication for their use in these illnesses since their effect is short-lived and there is a definite danger of addiction, with many dangerous side-effects.

Behaviour Therapy

In this type of treatment, which is still to some extent in the experimental stage, the patient is conditioned by means of carefully selected stimuli either to come to abhor some habit he wishes to lose or to tolerate some form of behaviour which he has previously been unable to enjoy.

Aversion therapy has been used with moderate success in the treatment of alcoholism: the patient is given alcohol and at the same time an injection which makes him violently sick, and by doing this repeatedly it may be possible to get him to associate a feeling of nausea with the thought of alcohol. Positive conditioning methods may be useful in, for example, phobic states: here the patient is helped to overcome the feared situation by gradually becoming used to it in a controlled fashion and by learning to employ relaxation techniques at times of anxiety.

New techniques are continually being devised in this form of treatment which is beginning to take a respectable place in the range of psychiatric therapies.

Hypnosis

Many lay people regard hypnosis as a near-magic form of treatment with dramatic curative effects. It rarely lives up to such expectations and in general its usefulness in psychiatry has proved very limited. Individuals who are readily hypnotizable and who are highly suggestible may gain symptomatic relief by direct suggestion given during a trance, but care has to be taken that suppression of symptoms does not intensify inner conflicts. However, hypnosis can sometimes be used to shorten the course of psychotherapy.

Other Forms of Psychological Treatment

We have not discussed the psychotherapies devised from the methods of Jung or Adler: small groups of disciples do practise psychological treatments based on their theories but their influence is relatively unimportant. There are innumerable other variations on the theme of psychotherapy: these include art therapy, music therapy and psychodrama. None of these is a true form of treatment, but may be of great help in engaging the interest and co-operation of particular patients. Relaxation therapy is widely used in hospitals and some individuals find that the learning of relaxation techniques can help them considerably at times of crisis and panic.

Other Forms of Physical Treatment

Psychotherapy with the aid of the drug L.S.D. is practised in some centres. This substance produces hallucinations and periods of confusion during which unconscious material may be released: later it may be of value to analyse this material with the patient. This is akin to abreaction techniques which are sometimes employed in acute neurotic illnesses: in this method the patient is given an injection of a quick-acting sedative drug and when his inhibitions are sufficiently in abeyance he is encouraged to express his fears and anxieties. In a successful treatment there is a dramatic emotional catharsis and a rapid release from anxiety.

Psychosomatic Illnesses

We are accustomed to think of mind and body as being separate entities, but there is very little justification for this theoretical division. Mental processes originate in the brain, which is a highly complex physical organ and which can be profoundly affected by events occurring in the body. Equally, thoughts and emotions can produce physical effects: happy anticipation can make the heart beat faster, anxiety can cause one to sweat and palpitate, depression can cause a number of physical processes to be slow and sluggish. Mind and body are inseparable in both health and illness and it is sometimes very difficult for a doctor to decide which element is predominant in a case of disease. Psychiatric patients often complain of somatic symptoms which seem very real to them and which may sometimes be accompanied by physical signs: the patient with anxiety neurosis does not imagine his increased pulse-rate. On the other hand, an individual's physical state can have repercussions on his frame of mind: we all know how miserable we feel when we have a severe stomach-ache and in some physical illnesses the patient may be precipitated into a true mental illness, as when influenza causes severe depression.

The term "Psychosomatic" (which simply means "mind-body") is used to describe this interaction of the mental and physical aspects of the organism. In medicine it is employed in two main ways. Firstly it indicates a general approach, drawing attention to the fact that there are important psychological and emotional factors which appear to precipitate or aggravate certain physical illnesses. Secondly, it is used to describe a group of physical illnesses in whose genesis emotional factors are considered to play an important part.

Some illnesses are almost entirely physical in origin and the patient's mental state has little influence in their causation. Many of the infectious illnesses come into this category (though it is worth noting that there is some evidence that conditions like the common cold are more likely to occur when a person is depressed). There are other somatic ailments in which psychological factors seem to play a much more important part and these are regarded as the psychosomatic illnesses. At various times enthusiasts have tried to incriminate emotional influence in the aetiology of virtually every physical disease and their uncritical approach has sometimes caused a certain amount of ridicule. Nowadays the ailments which are most commonly regarded as belonging to the psychosomatic category are asthma, peptic ulcer, ulcerative colitis, hypertension, migraine, coronary artery disease, pre-menstrual tension and some skin conditions. (Textbooks often list many more conditions than these: for example, dysmenorrhoea is usually quoted as a psychosomatic disorder though modern research has demonstrated that it is a "normal" complaint which occurs in a very high proportion of women.) It has been pointed out by a number of people that most of the illnesses accepted as being psychosomatic are also those which have a strong hereditary element. It seems possible that patients who develop psychosomatic illnesses have some inborn constitutional defect which breaks down under severe stress and results in the illness: this idea largely stems from Adler's theory of *Organ Inferiority*. Adler suggested that if some part of the body was markedly weaker than the rest, the entire organism would strive to compensate for this deficiency. Usually this process of compensation is valuable, as when a man with crippled legs strengthens his arms to increase his mobility, but sometimes it goes too far and the individual "over-compensates" for his disability. Thereafter his aims and drives become neurotically determined and the stress which this generates may lead to too much pressure on the mind or on the weak organ, with consequent psychiatric or psychosomatic illness. There is probably some element of truth in this hypothesis and we shall mention shortly how it has been adapted to modern knowledge.

There is no doubt that emotion can produce very marked physical changes and this has been demonstrated by numerous experiments in both animals and man. Extreme frustration has been shown to produce peptic ulcers in dogs and similar ulcers can also be produced by direct electrical stimulation of the portion of the brain known as the hypothalamus. Situations which cause overwhelming fear in rats can cause them to die as a result of acute failure of their adrenal glands: this may be analogous to the cases of death by witchcraft which are reported from various primitive peoples. It is of course not possible to carry out such severe experiments in human beings, but there have been opportunities at times to record the effects of emotion on the functions of inner organs: for example, there are some individuals who need to have a gastrostomy (an artificial opening into the stomach) because the gullet has become blocked for some reason and their stomach-lining can be directly observed while various pleasing or provocative psychological stimuli are presented to them. From these experiments it is known that the stomach reacts in characteristic ways to fear, pain, pleasure and other emotions just as that other organ, the skin, similarly reacts by blanching, blushing or perspiring. Many other organs are equally reactive to psychological stimuli and it is possible with modern physiological techniques to show, for example, that the blood flow in the coronary arteries changes during a stress-interview, that the concentration of various chemical substances in the blood alters with emotional events and that the blood clots more rapidly in an individual who is very anxious. (Some of these observations have been carried out on students waiting to sit an examination!) All of these changes suggest that if a stress is severe enough or prolonged enough there may eventually be overtaxing of the body's defences and subsequent breakdown into illness. There is also some evidence that emotional disorder can cause a delay in the disappearance of physical manifestations of illness: for example, it has been found that pneumonia takes longer to clear up in emotionally disturbed individuals than in normals, and presumably this represents another type of interference with physical defences.

We have been talking a good deal about stress, but what is psychological stress? It is difficult to generalize overmuch about this because everyone has his own particular stresses and breaking points. What is disturbing to someone may be quite neutral to someone else. One individual may find responsibility intolerable but be quite unworried by debt; another may be anxious all the time about money but be quite unmoved by physical danger; yet another may be able to face lions and tigers with equanimity but be terrified by mice or spiders. It was thought possible at one time that a particular type of stress could produce a specific physical illness, but this theory proved quite untenable. Then it was suggested that a particular personality structure would cause the individual to react to difficulties in a definite way: it was postulated that there was a "coronary thrombosis type" who was typically an over-ambitious and hard-driving executive, and a "peptic ulcer type" who reacted to habitual insecurity by being tense and over-perfectionistic. Careful studies have not confirmed these theories of personality specificity and nowadays the tendency is to believe that each emotional reaction has its own specific pattern of response within the autonomic nervous system (the part of the nervous system dealing with internal bodily functions). Under stress there may be over-activity of the nervous supply to some organ which will eventually become deranged in function. According to this theory it is a portion of the nervous system which may malfunction because of inborn abnormalities, but otherwise the hypothesis closely resembles that of Adler which we have mentioned previously. The autonomic nervous system is under the control of the hypothalamus and it is interesting that neurosurgeons have reported that peptic ulcer is not uncommon following intra-cranial operations when this part of the brain has been unavoidably over-stimulated: this finding is very similar to the results of animal experiments we have already noted and indicates how at least one physical disease can arise as a result of influences arising in the nervous system.

In general terms a psychosomatic illness can often be regarded as the unfortunate by-product of a process by which the body is attempting to protect itself against adverse influences. Some of these influences may be psychological and their effects are mediated through the brain and autonomic nervous system. The body has a natural tendency to maintain a state of equilibrium in all its systems and any influence which upsets this balance will call into play numerous self-righting mechanisms, both physical and psychological. If the struggle to regain equilibrium is too severe these mechanisms may no longer be effective and disease may result, the weakest part giving way first.

In addition to there being a connection between emotional stress and some physical illnesses there also appears to be an association between actual mental disorder and physical disease. Some people show an excessive tendency to develop a variety of both mental and physical illnesses and many normal people appear to go through phases in their lives when they are particularly liable to become ill, both physically and psychologically: for example, the menopausal period in women is notorious for this. In such cases it is often impossible to know whether one illness is the cause of the other or whether there is some unknown underlying factor present which renders the patient more likely to develop any sort of disease for a time. The picture is complicated by the presence of numerous other factors which can apparently influence the frequency of psychosomatic disorders. These illnesses appear most commonly between adolescence and middle age, they affect women rather more than men, they seem to be more frequent in urban than in rural areas, and they differ in frequency according to race and social class. In practice it is difficult to gather accurate data on psychosomatic conditions and the statistics we have are most unreliable, so many of our views on psychosomatic disorders must remain tentative. Further difficulties arise inasmuch as personality factors may influence illness patterns by means of such variables as diet, exercise, smoking, the drinking of alcohol and the taking of drugs.

We are forced to admit that our knowledge of psychosomatic factors remains vague and confusing but there is no doubt that the psychosomatic approach to illness in general has had markedly beneficial results. It has stressed that it is illogical to treat a disease without considering the man who is suffering from it. If an individual is emotionally disturbed or psychiatrically ill he may make physical complaints which have little or no organic basis and it is vital that the true nature of the condition be appreciated before inappropriate physical treatments are applied. If a patient is frustrated or unhappy his physical illness will often be more severe than it should be or it may respond less well than expected to treatment, and in this case recovery cannot be regarded as complete until the psychological element is also dealt with. The growing realization in various branches of medicine of the importance of social and psychological factors in the aetiology of physical disease has been one reason why the need for social work has come to be more generally accepted. Nowadays many illnesses need a multidisciplinary approach in order to heal the patient completely and the social worker can be regarded as a very important part of this therapeutic team. It would, therefore, be wise for every social worker to keep the "whole man" in view and never to let her own specialized work obscure other factors, either physical or psychological, which can only be ignored at the peril of impairing the patient's chances of full recovery.

Anorexia Nervosa

We have not mentioned this condition until now because it is easier to present it after having discussed the concept of psychosomatic illness. We do not regard anorexia nervosa as a true-psychosomatic condition but it certainly does occupy a borderland between mental and physical disease. Its name means "nervous lack of appetite" and the condition is characterized by the patient's extreme disinclination to eat, which naturally results in severe weight loss. Partial forms are not uncommon in young women who diet over-strenuously in order to be fashionably slim, but these are rarely considered as cases of illness. The more severe forms are not very frequent, but they constitute a problem which is quite out of proportion to their numbers as they tend to spend long periods in hospital and often require a great deal of social support following their discharge. The loss of appetite is psychological in origin, but anorexia nervosa cannot be considered as a separate psychiatric illness: it is an occasional symptom of a number of psychiatric disorders, notably obsessional neurosis, hysteria and schizophrenia, and it may also occur intermittently in some depressive patients. It appears predominantly in young women and at first it is often mistaken for some form of wasting physical disease: menstruation usually ceases and very severe constipation is common, but such physical symptoms are secondary to the severely restricted diet.

The condition usually begins in the teens or early twenties and often appears to start with the patient worrying about being over-weight, though the obesity may be evident only to herself. She then begins to diet and after a time the dieting gets out of control. Her weight goes down and down until she is almost skeletal in appearance but she herself appears content with her grotesque appearance. Her whole life revolves round food, or rather the refusal of it, and she takes just enough to keep alive but no more. In a few cases the patient actually does eat large amounts of food but regurgitates or vomits it as soon as it has been swallowed: some of these indivi-duals actually seem to enjoy vomiting as much as eating. The anorexic regards normal people as being obese and ugly and is anguished at the thought of becoming like them. She actively avoids attempts to increase her weight, either refusing to eat or else pretending to eat and then showing remarkable cunning in the hiding and dis-posing of the food. Physically she is weak and easily tired, but frequently she tries to maintain an impression of activity though this tends to be sporadic and often rather aimless.

A number of theories have been proposed to account for anorexia nervosa, but there is still disagreement as to the origin of the illness. Many of the patients are very immature sexually and it may be that starvation is their only way of coping with sexual impulses since by remaining very underweight all the emotions are kept much more feeble than normal. Whenever the weight begins to go up the emotions reassert themselves, which the patient finds extremely threatening, so she resists all attempts to fatten her. One psycho-analytic explanation of anorexia nervosa relates the symptoms to a severe degree of oral fixation in which the sexual fantasies are infantile and include fears of becoming pregnant through oral impregnation. The intake of food is equated with these fears and to prevent "sexual" contamination food has to be avoided. It is often found that other members of the household are obsessed by food in various ways and sometimes there are fads in the family eating habits which have laid the basis for the patient's trouble. The patient's initial worry about being overweight seems to act mostly as a trigger mechanism to set off an illness which would probably have occurred anyway.

Treatment depends partly on the actual cause of the anorexia. Depressive or schizophrenic illnesses have to be treated by appropriate means before the appetite will begin to improve. When a neurotic problem underlies the illness an attempt has to be made to resolve it, usually with psychotherapy, but anorexic patients often show a complete resistance to the gaining of insight. Where the loss of weight is really severe there is a definite danger of the patient starving to death and she will require admission to hospital. Once in hospital she is usually treated with drugs to reduce anxiety and to improve appetite and a fairly authoritarian approach towards her feeding is taken initially. Close supervision is needed to make sure that she really does take her nutrition and if she fails to gain weight it is quite certain that she is managing to avoid eating her food. With fairly firm handling, however, it is often possible to obtain a rapid increase in her weight. Unfortunately, there is a high relapse rate once the individual leaves hospital and there is frequently a suspicion that she gains weight only for the purpose of being allowed to finish treatment as quickly as possible so that she can return to her old state when she gets home.

Milder cases of anorexia nervosa smoulder on for a long time, without doing too much harm, but the outlook in severe cases is quite a poor one. Paradoxically, the patient stands a better chance of recovery from the anorexia when the underlying condition is a severe psychosis since the disturbance of appetite usually disappears with improvement in the mental state following treatment. Anorexia due to a severe psychoneurotic conflict tends to be very resistant to treatment and this type of patient needs a great deal of supervision and encouragement in addition to specific therapy. Following discharge from hospital a social worker may be asked to provide this supervision. These patients usually have very severe dependency problems and an understanding but firm approach by the social worker may help them gradually to develop more mature relationships. This can be facilitated if the psychiatrist and social worker adopt a concerted plan of action towards the patient. The anorexic is usually a past mistress at the art of manipulation and it is very important not to let her get her own way by playing one therapist against the other. In some cases admission to hospital is needed each time the weight drops, but as much as possible it is desirable to prevent the patient's becoming dependent on hospital as she can easily develop a great liking for the invalid's role. Consequently the social worker should give her every encouragement to maintain her health so as to develop the independence of which so often the anorexic is afraid.

CHAPTER 6

The Personality Disorders and Psychosexual Disorders

The Personality Disorders

This is a heterogeneous group of disorders in which the basic personality is noticeably abnormal. There is considerable disagreement about whether they can be regarded as true illnesses since in many instances they are merely quantitative deviations from normal and these deviations may be diffuse and relatively non-specific. To some extent the diagnosis constitutes a value-judgement because in order to make it one has to pronounce on what is normal, which in our present state of knowledge is often remarkably difficult. If we are fairly average individuals we will inevitably tend to regard people like ourselves as normal and any people who differ markedly from us will seem abnormal. Thus an exceedingly intelligent or an exceedingly dull individual might well be considered abnormal by average standards though there are plenty of such people around who otherwise show no evidence of being unhealthy or of deviating from accepted standards of behaviour. In fact, intelligence is not usually taken into account in assessing whether or not a personality disorder is present, but when examining a patient who is of a different social class or intelligence level from himself the clinician may sometimes be misled into thinking that these differences are really signs of illness.

The "average man" is a statistical myth, and in so far as we deviate psychologically in one way or another from the notional mean we all suffer from personality abnormalities. In the great majority of instances the deviation, whatever it is, is perfectly acceptable and neither the person nor society is any worse off for its existence. However, in some people a particular facet of personality is obviously very different from what can be accepted as normal or else the whole personality is distorted in some way. This does not necessarily imply the presence of an illness and, for example, a musical or mathematical prodigy may be considered as abnormal in this way and yet be highly valued nevertheless. But when someone is "different" there is a tendency for him to become isolated, and if his behaviour is at all odd this tendency may be increased. If he is difficult or aggressive he may come to be regarded as dangerous or, in an enlightened society, sometimes as ill. The fact of his being different often causes *him* a great deal of unhappiness and the more abnormal the personality the more likely is the person to break down into some form of psychiatric illness. When this happens he is doubly handicapped, firstly by his basic character disorder and secondly by the super-added illness. At times this illness is relatively distinct from the personality abnormality, but at other times it is mostly a further exaggeration of the already aberrant psychological state. The relative instability of individuals with personality disorders means that they often come to psychiatric attention. Obviously, the psychiatrist tends to see the most severe conditions of this type, but in the general population there are many people with milder forms of disorder which do not require treatment but are in nowise qualitatively different from the serious disorders.

Personality disorders often begin at an early age and there may well be a history of neurotic or difficult behaviour during childhood. Depending on the type of abnormality these childhood difficulties may manifest as excessive quietness, restlessness, aggressiveness or even delinquency. These features tend to become much more obvious around the time of puberty and in these people adolescence is often a highly explosive phase. Thereafter, in severely unstable cases there may be repeated exacerbations of neurotic or antisocial behaviour. Not infrequently there is a marked degree of inadequacy in social performance (which is not necessarily related to lack of intelligence) and this may appear in the form of lack of consistency and drive, poor interpersonal relationships, an unstable work record, brushes with authority and so on. But not all individuals with personality disorders are social failures and some may manage to compensate fairly successfully for their disabilities.

In most cases the reason for the personality disorder can only be guessed. In comparatively mild instances it simply represents a relative exaggeration or diminution of a normal facet of the character. In more serious examples there is often a history of a disturbed early upbringing and lack of consistent parental care and these seem to be important aetiological influences. At other times there is evidence of mild brain damage having occurred in early life, producing a certain degree of cerebral instability. Other notable aetiological factors include firstly being brought up in a delinquent household where emphasis is laid on antisocial values, and secondly the effect of heredity. This latter may have some importance since certain personality disorders such as psychopathy certainly seem to run in families. Some normal individuals who receive a head injury or suffer from encephalitis in adult life may undergo a marked character change and develop a very typical personality disorder. Whatever the cause of the condition, in many instances the manifestations are typically those of failure of maturation of the personality. In the milder case maturity can be attained though this is delayed, but in the more severe case the disorder remains present throughout life and its features are often further exaggerated by the onset of old age.

Numerous attempts have been made to classify the personality disorders, but these have not met with notable success. They are often such diffuse conditions that they elude close definition and they rarely possess characteristics which are exclusive to a particular type of disorder. We have not attempted to adhere to any theoretical principle of classification in describing them. Instead we have taken a number of widely accepted descriptive terms and we shall discuss in turn the illnesses to which they refer. It will soon become obvious that the features of many of the personality disorders closely resemble those of psychiatric illnesses we have described elsewhere, and for this reason they are sometimes known as character neuroses: but whereas most psychiatric illnesses come on after childhood and tend to be episodic, the personality disorders are habitual and usually unremitting. We shall tend to stress the associations between the two types of condition—for example, between the hysterical personality and hysteria, the schizoid personality and schizophrenia and so on. The majority of people with a personality disorder never break down into a psychiatric illness, but if they do, they often develop the illness which corresponds most closely with the prevailing character traits.

Before we describe the various disorders in detail we wish to mention two terms in common use. Many people talk about the "inadequate personality" as though it were a diagnosis but in fact it simply denotes someone who shows a general lack of nous and a tendency to lead a disorganized life. This may occur in association with a number of psychiatric conditions or may be seen in otherwise normal individuals and the term is used more often in an abusive sense than any other. Likewise, the "immature personality" is a vague concept which also has derogatory connotations, but at least when it is used it implies some failure of development which may possibly be remedied. Both terms are occasionally useful for descriptive purposes but should not be over-employed.

Let us now consider the main types of personality disorder in turn.

1. *The Anxious Personality*

A great many people in the general population will admit to being "nervous" or "highly strung" and yet despite this they appear to lead full and happy lives. They are often estimable citizens who do their best to please others, work hard in order to maintain a good name and are rather easily upset by criticism or harsh words, but their nervousness causes them relatively little discomfort. However, in some people of this type anxiety is more severe and is present so much of the time that it interferes with their ability to do certain things, to enjoy themselves or to relax thoroughly. The feeling of tension becomes even worse when extra responsibility has to be shouldered or when there is some threat to security. In the most serious cases it may become impossible to perform everyday tasks or take part in normal activities and attempts to do these things sometimes lead to attacks of panic. Allied to these difficulties there is often excessive shyness and sensitivity and as a result the person may find great difficulty in being at ease in company.

In some cases these feelings of anxiety increase till they come to dominate the patient's existence so that he is constantly afraid and unhappy. Agitation causes muscular tension and the resulting aches and pains may convince him that he is suffering from a variety of serious physical ailments. This leads him to become very hypochondriacal and as a result he may complain much more of physical than of mental discomfort. Every so often the symptoms may flare up into a full-blown anxiety state and quite frequently this is followed by a period of depression. Not uncommonly it is this depression which finally brings the person to psychiatric attention and it is striking to notice how often a depressive patient will admit to having been an excessive worrier prior to the onset of his illness. Despite the numerous complaints of poor physical health, most anxious individuals have no underlying somatic disease to account for their symptoms. But occasionally quite typical chronic anxiety can be caused by physical disease so it is always important to be certain that the possibility of this has been excluded when a diagnosis is being made.

Most anxious people do not require treatment for this particular trait if it remains within reasonable limits but if tension symptoms are excessively troublesome some form of psychiatric intervention may be necessary. It is always wise to look for any environmental difficulty such as domestic, interpersonal or work problems which may be aggravating the person's natural tendency to be anxious, and if this can be remedied life may become much more tolerable for him. Psychotherapy is sometimes required but this is usually more effective in dealing with the secondary emotional problems which have appeared as a consequence of the personality disorder. The disorder itself is often too fundamental to respond dramatically to psychological treatment. Tranquillizing drugs are useful but much less effective than in an acute anxiety state. The social worker may provide a valuable supportive influence for a patient with a chronically anxious personality since an understanding and calm approach may be as therapeutic as more formal types of treatment.

2. *The Depressive Personality*

This type of personality disorder is quite easily recognizable but rather difficult to define. We all know individuals who have a perpetual air of pessimism and defeatism and for whom life never seems to go well (at least according to them). Some of these people have a certain amount of insight into their attitudes and may even view them with a degree of wry humour, but often there is a grumbling, self-pitying air about them which irritates other people after a time. Hypochondriacal complaints are frequent and some of these chronically depressed individuals are indefatigable swallowers of patent medicines. As with all disorders of personality, the symptoms may never pass beyond this stage but episodes of frank depressive illness are comparatively common and at times there may be a good deal of anxiety admixed with the depression. This is often related to worries over health, but sometimes the anxiety symptoms appear to be autonomous and have no relation to actual circumstances. As with anxiety states, crises are poorly coped with and there is a tendency for the person to retreat from any sort of difficulty rather than make a decision or take some form of action.

It is important when seeing someone with what appears to be a depressive personality disorder not to miss an actual depressive illness. Some relatively mild depressive conditions may be very chronic and last for several years on end so that after a time the patient and his family come to accept the depression as the normal mood-state. Some of these cases respond well to antidepressant treatment and this should always be given if there is any chance that it will succeed, but in the true personality disorder the depressive symptoms usually respond only slightly to treatment. Psychotherapy, usually of the supportive type, may be helpful in dealing with some of the patient's neurotic problems. If practical help is required it mostly consists of aiding the patient to develop confidence and learn to make his own decisions. With some individuals it may eventually have to be recognized that their "Weary Willy"attitude is their only adequate defence against life's everyday problems and in the long run it may be safer to leave them with their depression and their constant grumbling.

3. *The Obsessional Personality*

In Chapter 5 we have discussed the main features of obsessional neurosis and have mentioned that this is an illness which often (though not invariably) arises in the setting of obsessional personality traits. We have pointed out that an obsessional stage is normal in the development of every young child and that in some instances the child does not fully outgrow the features of this stage and is left with noticeable traits of obsessionality in his personality. In the mildest cases these may hardly affect the person at all and may be regarded as normal and even desirable characteristics—for example, tidiness, punctuality and self-discipline. Sometimes it is the "magical element" of the obsessional stage which persists and then the person may be prone to indulge in superstitious beliefs and practices which have a ritual "undoing" effect. For instance, he may genuinely believe that touching wood or reciting a set phrase will enable him to avoid danger.

If the obsessional traits are stronger than this the individual may tend to be over-careful and to become unhappy if everything is not in its proper order. These perfectionistic tendencies are highly regarded by society and are necessary for certain occupations. One would prefer one's banker or accountant to be obsessional! However, when the traits are really powerful they may go beyond a desire for order and efficiency and may cause the person real discomfort and anxiety if he finds that he cannot control his environment. They are often accompanied by a severe rigidity of temperament which produces over-conformism, puritanism and an inability to adapt readily to changes. Many obsessional people are insecure in themselves and have difficulty in expressing their emotions. They are unable to show overt aggression and on the surface they often appear mild and anxious to agree, though in fact it is frequently only their firm control over their emotions which prevents anger from bursting out. The obsessional turns his feelings inwards and drives himself unrelentingly, denying himself pleasure in order to try to satisfy his unappeasable conscience. It is this severe type of obsessional personality in which tension symptoms are likely to appear and, in some cases, herald the gradual onset of an obsessional neurosis. These symptoms often occur after the person has incurred some extra responsibility such as marriage or promotion. The obsessional is also particularly apt to develop periods of depression because things affect him deeply and he is inclined to brood a great deal.

Psychoanalytic theory postulates that the individual with an obsessional personality has experienced a fixation of libido at the anal stage of emotional development and it describes the condition as the Anal Personality. This particular failure of emotional maturation is usually found in association with a harsh and over-zealous superego which views everything in terms of absolute right and wrong. But since an adult appreciates that he can never achieve complete rightness the obsessional is always falling short of the dictates of his conscience. There is little doubt about the over-stringency of the obsessional's superego, but it must be said that the theory regarding anal fixation is not universally accepted. It is possible that there is an hereditary factor present in the genesis of the obsessional personality as there is in obsessional neurosis. Certainly in some cases there is an underlying element of organic brain damage. This is seen very strikingly in old people, who tend to become excessively careful and who make up for failing intellectual powers by insisting on an unchanging series of routines in their everyday lives. Any attempt to disturb these routines is likely to result in the person's having a severe panic reaction.

Many obsessional people experience sexual difficulties. These may sometimes be due to an inhibited upbringing, causing an inculcated belief that sex is dirty or producing feelings of shyness with members of the opposite sex. Often there is a good deal of guilt about sexual thoughts and practices. If the individual finds it difficult to make contact with the opposite sex there may be a great deal of sexual fantasy and masturbation, resulting in guilt feelings and, at times, hypochondriacal worry about possible damage to the health. Occasionally the obsessional's repressive defences conceal a good deal of primitive and even sadistic sexual fantasy, but often the result of this is an overt display of sexual puritanism or else prurience concealed under a cloak of prudishness in the person who enjoys nosing out other people's peccadillos.

The mildly obsessional person who has found his niche in life is often a respected member of the community whose hard work and cautiousness are admired, and he rarely seems to progress to illness. It is the severe obsessional who is most likely to suffer from the ill-effects of his personality traits and who is liable to develop a true psychiatric illness. When he does develop such an illness he rarely makes society suffer as a result. His anguish is turned inwards and it is he who is unhappy, but he often conceals his troubles and tries to keep on when many others would have complained much earlier. However, the appearance of additional psychiatric symptoms eventually makes life intolerable for him and he is forced to seek help. When treatment is instituted it is often directed at the secondary psychiatric features such as tension or depression to begin with. Thereafter it may be possible to conduct some form of psychotherapy to enable the individual to adjust more comfortably to his everyday existence. Therapy involving deep insight is usually not feasible because the person's psychic defences are too rigid and he rarely becomes able to achieve true relaxation, most often remaining fussy and over-anxious. Any environmental problems which aggravate his tension should be dealt with if this is possible and if he is willing to co-operate. Tranquillizing drugs are useful in reducing his prevailing level of anxiety. Fortunately, in the course of time, many severely obsessional personalities appear to mellow, and though they often remain rigid and over-strict other traits become less bothersome.

4. *The Hysterical Personality*

In many ways this diagnosis is synonymous with that of immature personality. Much hysterical symptomatology is reminiscent of childish behaviour or of the behaviour of old people who are becoming childish. Most adults are capable of behaving in a regressive fashion if they are sufficiently frustrated. This tendency is increased under conditions of tiredness, physical debility or mental strain, but in normal circumstances behaviour is appropriate to the situation and such people are able to tolerate a good deal of uncertainty and anxiety. Individuals with hysterical personalities appear to have failed to develop a well-integrated adult personality and their behaviour is frequently unstable and unreliable. Superficially they usually appear perfectly normal, but their ability to withstand frustration is extremely limited and they over-react to every minor crisis which occurs.

Hysterical individuals display a great deal of emotion but this is usually superficial and inconsistent. Typically these people cannot form deep and lasting relationships with others. They are fond of proclaiming their undying affections until they are put to the test and then there is often a rapid retreat from the emotional involvement. The hysteric is excessively narcissistic and demands a great show of affection from others: in the absence of such demonstration she will demand attention and she does not mind stirring everyone else's feelings for her own satisfaction. Individual methods for gaining notice will vary from constant badgering, through sulks and tantrums, to dramatic "death-scenes" and even suicidal attempts (which are sometimes dangerous and even fatal though probably not intended to be so).

Underneath the show of immediate warmth and friendship hysterics are often emotionally infantile and sexually frigid. Their histrionic qualities and surface glitter can make them very attractive short-term acquaintances, but profoundly unsatisfying partners. The floridly hysterical personality is much commoner in women than in men. When these women marry they not infrequently become professional martyrs or invalids, dramatizing their inability to sustain a sexual relationship by proclaiming that the husband is unhealthily interested in sex or opting out of it on grounds of chronic ill-health. If they become mothers they are frequently over-possessive and use all their wiles to retain the child's affections exclusively for themselves, meanwhile proclaiming their goodness as mothers though in fact they receive much more from the relationship than they ever give.

It is always difficult to prevent a note of disapproval from creeping in when discussing hysterics, reprehensible though this may be. Often such people are merely immature and ineffectual but in some cases their proclivity for manipulating others' affairs can be positively malignant and their typical lack of insight makes it very difficult to reason or remonstrate with them. Some hysterics with stronger personalities may be able to put their characteristics to good use and, for example, their histrionic tendencies and ability to simulate emotion may make them very successful on the stage. In these circumstances they do well so long as they are enjoying acclaim, but whenever things go wrong they become anxious and are then likely to break down.

The most severe cases of hysterical personality disorder shade into other forms of psychiatric abnormality such as psychopathy and into various forms of antisocial behaviour such as confidence tricks and pathological lying. In a small number of cases the patient shows an unaccountable desire to enter hospital and undergo surgical operation. This last form of behaviour is characterized by the patient's ability to simulate severe pain and sometimes even to produce abnormal physical signs, and is often referred to as the "Münchausen syndrome" (after Baron Münchausen, a fictional character who blandly told the most outrageous lies about his career). It is not a separate type of psychiatric illness but is rather a sub-type of hysterical personality disorder. In some individuals it is linked with a desire to obtain drugs and these people often appear in casualty departments complaining very convincingly of agonizing pain in order to get an injection of morphine or similar substance. If his complaints are disregarded the patient may resort to the swallowing of pins, cutlery and other improbable articles in order to force the performing of an operation and the administration of drugs. Some of these people travel all over the country, using assumed names and obtaining countless admissions to hospital and many of them are criss-crossed with operation scars. For their own sakes these patients need psychiatric supervision and if a social worker ever suspects that she is dealing with an individual of this type she should immediately convey her suspicions to her medical colleagues. Nowadays, drug addiction is a growing problem and hysterics are a group who are particularly at risk. Many of them are flighty and easily led and they are ripe material for the drug-pedlar since they are often easily addicted.

Hysterical neuroses very often, though not invariably, develop out of an hysterical personality and they can usually be seen as exacerbations of the patient's prevailing personality traits. As with the person suffering from the neurosis, the individual with an hysterical personality shows a marked ability to defend herself by the psychological process of dissociation. Cerebral function tends to be less stable than normal, and under stress psychological elements which are proving too unpleasant to be borne are blocked from consciousness and either transferred completely to another psychological compartment or apparently converted to physical symptoms. Psychological testing confirms that hysterical individuals are basically more neurotic and more suggestible than normal.

The aetiology of the hysterical personality is probably related to a number of factors. By using the electroencephalogram it is possible to demonstrate that the hysterical tendencies are associated with a lack of brain maturation in some patients. In others it may be a result of actual brain damage which has occurred before or after birth and which is something associated with epilepsy. In the majority of hysterics there is no direct evidence of abnormal brain function but there is frequently a history of some disturbance in their upbringing; in particular, there has often been lack of proper emotional warmth in the relationship with the parents, perhaps due to parental coldness, a broken home or the lack of stable parent-figures. In circumstances like these the child does not receive sufficient emotional attention to enable normal affective development to take place; she has to demand love and if this is not forthcoming she will demand any other kind of show of emotion to the point of rousing anger. This becomes habitual and the individual remains demanding but always unsatisfied. In boys the demands may come to be associated with aggression and this may result in psychopathic behaviour, but in girls it is commoner for the emotions to remain child-like. According to psychoanalytic theory there is fixation at an oral stage of libidinal development and it is suggested that this has usually been due to some disturbance of the Oedipal situation. This formulation appears to hold true for only a minority of hysterics.

Most hysterical individuals do not need treatment for their personality abnormality. If psychiatric treatment is required it is usually for a superadded neurotic illness or for one of the pathological complications of hysteria such as the Münchausen syndrome. If the patient's complaints are caused by anxiety-provoking situations or interpersonal difficulties it is usually simpler to deal with these than to treat the patient, mainly because of her resistance to insight. A mixture of superficial supportive psychotherapy, direct suggestion and practical help is the usual prescription. The social worker is often called upon to provide the support in these cases and she can be a tower of strength provided that she is able to resist demands to become involved in all the patient's little emotional crises and provided also that she can tolerate frequent accusations of ill-faith and lack of concern, the hysteric's weapons against supposed indifferences. It is important to be able to accept such childish tantrums and not be tempted to reply in kind. To help the patient you must be more mature than she, though carefully avoiding any hint of condescension. At times the social worker's intervention is as helpful to the family as it is to the patient herself since they are often emotionally worn out by the frequent outbursts. Fortunately hysterical personalities tend to mature in time, even if in many cases the maturity is just sufficient to enable the person to become a tolerable, though still difficult, member of the community. By providing a stable influence the social worker may possibly hasten this process.

5. *The Cycloid Personality*

We are all subject to swings of mood, but these are normally neither too severe nor too prolonged. However, there are some people who are particularly liable to become elated or depressed without any obvious reason and they are said to have a cycloid or cyclothymic personality because their moods show a tendency to occur in cycles. Such individuals sometimes get a reputation for being "moody" because they are so changeable: people tend to notice the episodes of depression and irritability, but may not be nearly so aware of the periods of upswing. In mild forms this type of personality is relatively common and is in no way to be regarded as an illness, but the more severe forms do show an excessive tendency to develop manic-depressive disorders in some cases. It is said that people with cycloid personalities are to be found commonly among the relatives of manic-depressives and it has been suggested that the abnormality is a partial form of that illness and due to the same (presumed) genetic influences.

Most often the cyclothymic individual does not require psychiatric treatment, though he may sometimes complain that his frequent changes of mood interfere with his efficiency at work or with his personal relationships. It is quite common for a social worker to meet with such people when dealing with the families of manic-depressive patients. It is worth noting the presence of the abnormality since it is a useful diagnostic pointer towards the prevailing type of mental disorder in the family. It is also worth identifying the individual as being potentially at risk of developing the same illness as his relative: this would not be an indication for instituting treatment but rather a point of information for the future lest the person did become ill.

6. *The Schizoid Personality*

Just as the cycloid personality appears to have a relationship with manic-depressive illness, so the schizoid personality is often found in the relatives of schizophrenics and may occur in some schizophrenics prior to the actual onset of their illness. Also, just as many cyclothymics never develop manic-depressive disorders, so the majority of people with schizoid traits are not schizophrenic and will never develop this illness. Nevertheless it has been suggested that well-marked forms of this personality disorder are genetically related to schizophrenia. Typically the schizoid individual is somewhat shy, aloof and withdrawn. He tends to prefer his own company and to be ill-at-ease socially. He avoids prominence and sometimes his existence becomes almost hermit-like. Often he is rather humourless and over-sensitive to criticism, tending to brood on slights and to magnify their significance. At times his asocial behaviour reaches the point of eccentricity and he may gain a reputation as a crank or a fanatic, particularly if he has a penchant for belonging to strange societies or esoteric religious groups.

We can probably pick out quite readily from our acquaintances someone who fulfils a number of these criteria but who is nevertheless reasonably well adjusted, and the great majority of shy and sensitive people are not psychologically disturbed. However, the schizoid relative of a schizophrenic patient should be noted as someone who may be at risk.

A schizoid individual often has considerable difficulty in expressing emotion and may be excessively wrapped up in his own interests. If he is married his aloofness may make for difficulties between him and his spouse and children. A schizoid mother may be unable to provide her children with a normal amount of emotional warmth and may be cool and unsympathetic when they are distressed or in pain. The result of this may be an emotionally deprived child who exhibits behaviour disorders, and if he is genetically predisposed to schizophrenia he may be precipitated into the illness by the behaviour of his so-called "schizophrenogenic" mother. Perhaps fortunately the severe schizoid shows a pronounced tendency to remain unmarried, which at least means fewer disturbed children but on the other hand tends to increase his isolation. A schizoid individual often has little wish to change his way of life, but it may be important to prevent him from becoming more and more asocial and the social work approach may be more effective than formal treatment in this. Often it is even more important to ensure that members of his family receive help or treatment if they are suffering from the effects of his emotional coldness.

7. *The Paranoid Personality*

This disorder often appears to be related to the schizoid personality but there is usually less withdrawal and more touchiness. The paranoid individual is over-sensitive and may be convinced that he is being deliberately victimized by others. Since he is quite frequently a rather eccentric person his suspicions are sometimes justified. His odd behaviour tends to antagonize people or make him distrusted and as a result he may well fail to get on as well as he should at work and in his social milieu. Since he is likely to lack adequate insight into his own limitations and idiosyncrasies he tends to rationalize his lack of success by attributing it to the malice of other people. He may imagine that they dislike him because of some feature of his appearance or because he belongs to a religious minority or because he is too clever for them. At first these self-justifications are some compensation for failure, but eventually he is liable to become embittered. When this happens he may either brood endlessly over the supposed wrongs done to him or else he complains endlessly and ineffectually to whoever will listen.

Not all paranoid individuals are so inadequate. In certain cases the person is quite likely to take some kind of action in order to voice his protest. This is the sort of individual who is extremely touchy and nettles at every wrong, whether real or imagined. He guards his rights jealously and at times he may be socially useful as a kind of citizen's watchdog if his complaints are just, because he is usually the first to complain over any infringement of liberty. Unfortunately he is often as much a nuisance as a benefit to his cause since his excessive complaining and needless irritability tend to alienate support. Sometimes such people gain minor prominence in some struggle over bureaucratic interference, but frequently they lose sympathy because their dissatisfaction is never appeased. A number of them become litigious and drag their cases through the law courts, never accepting defeat as such and always claiming that they were the victims of a legal miscarriage. Others become chronic hypochondriacs, convinced that they have some serious disease and going from one specialist to another, never believing a negative verdict and ignoring the obvious fact that they have been complaining for so long that a potentially fatal illness would have killed them long ago.

Many individuals with paranoid personality traits can manage to exist reasonably well despite their constant belief of ill-usage, but in others the struggle against real and imaginary difficulties can cause periods of anxiety or depression which may require treatment. It may be difficult to give adequate psychiatric treatment because some of these patients readily come to believe that the psychiatrist is also against them. In some cases the person eventually becomes frankly deluded and even hallucinated and then breaks down into a true paranoid schizophrenia. The onset of the illness may seem to have been precipitated by a particular event, but in many cases it has actually been developing for a considerable time beforehand.

It is rarely pleasant or easy to deal with a patient who has a paranoid personality and it is as well to realize how difficult he may be. One must be sympathetic with him if he is ill and has troubles, but it is essential not to be persuaded to side with him in his unfounded complaints. It is quite useless in most cases to try to argue sense into him when his grievances are obviously unfounded. When he proves unusually obstructive or difficult it is advisable to consult with your psychiatrist colleague regarding the management of the case, otherwise you may find yourself involved in some extremely tangled situation of the patient's making.

8. *The Affectionless Personality*

This type of disorder is probably a sub-category of psychopathy, but it does not necessarily produce antisocial behaviour and it sometimes seems to have an affinity with the schizoid personality. The individual appears to lack most of the finer feelings and he is relatively unaware of emotions such as sympathy, affection and compassion. He often seems to have little need of human company, but his lack of emotional warmth may be covered by a superficial layer of bonhomie which is sufficient to persuade people who do not know him very well that he is perfectly normal. Such a personality abnormality can be quite compatible with a successful career since, if the person has drive and ability, he can make straight for his goal without being diverted by normal emotional needs. As well as this, he is quite prepared to use other people ruthlessly for his own ends without feeling particular remorse if this does them harm. As may be imagined, such an individual is rarely popular and if he or she marries the partner is frequently unhappy because of this lack of human feeling. The affectionless person does not suffer as a result of this, but quite often the spouse breaks down under the strain of the non-relationship. The cause of this breakdown is often not obvious to others because of the veneer of normality and respectability assumed by the other partner, but when the psychiatrist or social worker has to deal with him as the relative of a patient his emotional coldness and arrogance often become apparent. It is usually impossible to persuade him to change his attitudes because he is unmoved by the distress he causes to others.

The affectionless personality seems to arise most often in those who have been very severely emotionally deprived in early childhood. The typical history is of parental coldness or cruelty, a severely disturbed early home or an institutional upbringing. There appears to be a more or less complete failure of development of the higher emotions though sometimes this is more noticeable in one area of the personality than in another. For example, some of these people can show no affection for individual human beings yet may become passionately involved in excellent causes. Sometimes the individual has relatively normal sexual appetites, though usually using the opposite sex for enjoyment without concern for the feelings of others. In other cases there is either very little sexual emotion or, as is not at all uncommon, various forms of sexual perversion.

Despite the affectionless person's apparent self-sufficiency he is, in common with all possessors of personality disorders, more than normally liable to develop some form of psychiatric disorder. Various types of neurotic and hypochondriacal complaints are relatively frequent and suicide is quite often a feature of the condition. This last is sometimes related to a flash of insight when the individual appears to realize how empty his life is and in a mood of self-disgust tries to end it. In our experience the suicidal affectionless person is one who is very likely to kill himself and who is extremely difficult to dissuade from this course.

Obviously if the affectionless personality is combined with

other features of psychopathy or criminality the result may be a highly dangerous antisocial individual. We shall discuss this aspect later when we deal with the Callous Psychopath (see p. 140).

Psychopathy

Up till now, most of the abnormalities of personality we have been describing are fairly readily acceptable as illnesses, especially in their extremer forms when the patient is often tense and unhappy and is unable to enjoy normal social relationships. But in this section of the book we have to discuss a condition in which the individual usually appears to suffer very little, if at all, from his abnormality but may frequently make other people suffer as a result of his conduct. The psychopath is often actively antisocial rather than just asocial and in fact he is sometimes called a sociopath because of this strong tendency to clash with the rules of society. He presents innumerable problems to psychiatrists and legal authorities alike, including the vexed question (which it would be unprofitable to go into here) of just how responsible he is for his disordered behaviour. However, there is little doubt that the psychopath does show evidence of psychological disturbance and, as we shall mention, because he is particularly liable to develop other forms of psychiatric disorders we have no hesitation in presenting this as a psychiatric condition, while stressing the presence of numerous sociolegal complications.

The psychopath is an individual who shows an abnormal degree of egocentricity and who has little or no capacity for feeling remorse when he has done something wrong. He has no more than a superficial appreciation of rightness and wrongness and fails to learn from experience as other people do. His conduct is therefore little altered by either punishment or kindness. A capacity for foresight is conspicuous by its absence so that behaviour is rarely determined by fear of its consequences. Complete lack of conscience is often coupled with irresponsibility and foolhardiness and when these are associated with antisocial trends the result is likely to be a dangerous and unpredictable criminal. Most criminals are not particularly psychopathic, but the ones who are form a highly explosive minority.

Psychopaths often behave in such an irrational fashion that they appear to be intellectually retarded, but mental deficiency is not a particular feature of their disorder. There are indeed psychopaths who are dull, but the majority are of normal intelligence and a number are of above average ability. Many of them present a superficial appearance of normality and some (as we have described in the Affectionless Personalities) can disguise their abnormalities sufficiently to lead a normal-seeming life. If the disorder is of any degree of severity at all it usually expresses itself in some way and most psychopaths lead an erratic and disordered life, at least in their earlier years. They have no consistent goals at which to aim and almost invariably they grab at immediate pleasure and gratification instead of holding towards longer-term objectives. They are utterly unreliable people and may be pathological liars, who are sometimes very convincing at first but who usually are unable to avoid contradicting their own lies after a time. Some of them are adept at giving an appearance of trust-worthiness but this is a façade. Basically they are shiftless, insincere and quite capable of any form of cheating and dishonesty. They are perfectly unashamed of their ability to deceive people and it is essential that the social worker, when dealing with a psychopath, should know that he is almost always out for his own ends and will lie, flatter, cajole or threaten in order to gain them. If he is a patient he will co-operate for just so long as it suits him, but whenever the act becomes too tedious or some temptation appears he will quickly revert to his habitual misdeeds.

No matter how normal his appearance and behaviour appear on the surface the individual with a severely psychopathic personality is one of the most abnormal people in the community, and with his aggressiveness and lack of any moral sensibility he can also be one of the most dangerous. Yet, most of the time his behaviour is not psychotic and many inexperienced people are unable to believe that an apparently average person can be as utterly unreliable and criminous as many psychopaths are. The social worker must not be naïve in her attitude to the psychopath. She must be aware of his capacity for gulling and cheating others and should realize that repeated experience has shown that when a social worker attempts a personal crusade to reform a psychopath, more often than not he remains unchanged and the social worker is left looking foolish or even suffers personal damage. In order to help a psychopath one must refuse to enter his shiftless frame of reference and always the attempt should be to persuade him to accept the values of normal society, for something which he is very unlikely to show much willingness.

We have been referring to the psychopath throughout as "he" and it is true that the majority of severe psychopaths are males. There are many female psychopaths, but their behaviour is usually a great deal less aggressive than that of the men and in many instances it is difficult to distinguish them from those women who display the typical acting-out of the hysterical personality.

The late Sir David Henderson classified psychopaths into three main types. Nowadays his classification is often criticized, but it is still widely employed and we shall use it as a convenient framework within which to discuss the concept of the condition. Henderson described psychopaths as being predominantly *Aggressive, Inadequate* or *Creative*. In the aggressive and inadequate forms the basic abnormalities are similar, but the aggressive psychopath is much more liable to outbursts of temper and violence whereas the inadequate psychopath is characterized rather by instability, fecklessness and non-violent forms of law-breaking. In fact the two forms are not distinct and many individuals are inadequate at one time and aggressive at another. The creative group is one whose existence is not accepted by many people, but it is certainly true that many very prominent people have unusual and even abnormal personalities. In some instances the abnormality may have contributed to their rise to fame, and even where the abnormality is essentially psychopathic these people may still be capable of making some contribution to society. For example, we would imagine that a number of famous artists have been psychopathic and certainly some of them have shown little concern for the values of society, yet their work may now be widely admired. The same may be said about a proportion of prominent political figures and business tycoons. If it seems too extreme to label such individuals as psychopaths, perhaps it would be more acceptable to include them in the group of affectionless personality disorders we have already described.

The aggressive psychopath is someone who, apart from his other personality abnormalities, is unstable and is readily provoked to anger or may have spontaneous outbursts of rage. When these outbursts are very violent and appear without undue provocation, the condition is sometimes known as Explosive Psychopathy. Before a rage there is often a period of moodiness when the individual is more than usually irritable. Then a small incident sparks off his temper or else he sets out to pick a quarrel or start a fight. Afterwards he shows no concern about any harm he may have done and even if he has caused serious injury or even committed murder his only real concern is for the safety of his own skin. There is no feeling of regret or pity towards the victim and the psychopath's lack of insight and his endless capacity for self-justification soon convince him that he was really the injured party. Psychopaths make completely unreliable witnesses whether or not they have been responsible for an offence. When they take up a criminal career, as many of them do, they are often feared and disliked by other criminals because of their unpredictability and needless violence. Their uncertain tempers are often made worse by excessive drinking and sometimes they exhibit grossly abnormal behaviour under the influence of alcohol. Sooner or later a considerable number of psychopaths become chronic alcoholics and, at the present time, drug addiction is a growing problem, especially among the younger psychopaths.

The majority of psychopaths are heterosexual, but, like his other emotions, his sexual drive tends to be crude and to demand instant gratification. He rarely has true affection for a sexual partner and if he marries he is often irresponsible and cruel towards his wife and children. Because he lacks forethought he often neglects contraceptive precautions and produces a series of unwanted pregnancies. Sexual perversions are common, and if they are combined with severe aggressiveness they may lead to sexual crimes and even murder. Some sexual psychopaths actively enjoy killing and torturing, and obtain sexual pleasure from doing this. If they escape the consequences of their first misdeed they may repeat it again and again. This tendency to recidivism is frequently seen in whatever form of crime the psychopath has turned to, and attempts to reform and rehabilitate the young psychopathic individual often fail. The less intelligent criminal psychopath may be fairly easily caught after his first offence because of his over-confidence and his failure to take precautions against detection. The cleverer psychopath can compensate on an intellectual level for his emotional abnormalities and may make an extremely astute and pitiless law-breaker.

The inadequate psychopath may be a person who simply drifts along, forever cadging and always taking the easiest way out of his difficulties but never doing much positive harm. On the other hand, he may be the less competent type of criminal, the petty thief, confidence trickster or small-time swindler. He lives on his wits and sometimes displays a talent for making easy money: usually his talent for spending or losing it is even greater. Sometimes these people develop grandiose ideas about their own capabilities and start ambitious business projects which are backed by gullible members of the public. Most often their schemes crash, but this never deters a psychopath for long and he is soon engaged on another ill-fated scheme. He shows no real regret at any hardship he may cause others as a result of his activities and it is remarkable how often he escapes the real consequences of his misdeeds by his glibness and superficial charm. This charm readily disappears when he is forced into a corner and then he may display a good deal of aggression and even violence.

All psychopaths lack the ability to empathize with other human beings and their relationships with most people are shallow but extremely demanding. Nevertheless, they occasionally show a partial ability to take part in a two-sided emotional relationship. In one sub-group of the psychopathic personalities, the so-called *Callous Psychopath,* the individual appears to possess no normal feelings whatsoever. He is not always overtly aggressive, but he has absolutely no pity and he may take a perverted delight in cold-blooded cruelty. This type of man makes the ideal torturer or assassin, but his lack of human responsiveness is so uncanny that his allies are often as afraid of him as his enemies. Such grossly abnormal people are not frequently met with but they do exist and are highly dangerous.

Partial forms of psychopathy are relatively common and are not usually considered as psychiatric problems, but severely psychopathic individuals frequently come to psychiatric attention as a result of their personality disorder or one of its complications. Since they usually lead thoroughly disorganized lives their affairs are often chaotic. When they are young this rarely bothers them very much, but eventually a proportion of them develop anxiety symptoms and hypochondriasis is also quite common. In the rather older psychopath, depression is fairly frequent and may be very severe in some cases. Some of these patients develop an extremely profound degree of self-disgust, as though insight had dawned and was too painful to bear, and they may go out of their way to seek dangerous situations or actively try to kill themselves. This is particularly so when alcoholism or drug addiction is also a severe problem.

In most instances the psychopath has displayed abnormalities of behaviour from a very early age. As a child he often distinguishes himself by lying, thieving, disobedience and bullying. He may run away from home repeatedly or be thoroughly irresponsible in various ways. With the onset of puberty his difficult behaviour becomes much more obvious and his antisocial activities more serious. This pattern is not invariable and in a certain number of cases where the adult behaviour is typically psychopathic there is a history of a normal childhood and then subsequently a severe change of personality. Most often this is due to the effects of a head injury or of encephalitis, but sometimes it would appear that a schizophrenic illness has appeared and then, for some reason, halted at an early stage.

What do we know about the actual causation of psychopathy? In the first place we know enough to realize that it is not a single illness entity. The psychopathic personality may be the end-product of a number of abnormal influences. One of the most important of these is a disturbed early upbringing, particularly where there has been a marked degree of emotional deprivation, parental rejection or cruelty. However, the majority of emotionally deprived children do not grow up to be psychopathic and it is not at all clear why they escape unharmed. A good many psychopaths have not had abnormal upbringings, or at least if their childhood background was abnormal this was because their personality disorder was already there to cause trouble. Some cases of this type show evidence of abnormal brain-function as measured by the E.E.G. (electro-encephalogram) and often the brain-disturbance is essentially a failure of maturation. This corresponds well with the individual's behaviour, which typically displays the self-centredness of the young child. Evidence is emerging at the present time that certain specific abnormalities of the sex-chromosomes may be the basic cause of the abnormal behaviour in another small group of criminal psychopaths. Explosive psychopaths are quite commonly found to be suffering from a form of epilepsy and their disturbed behaviour may improve markedly when they are given anticonvulsant drugs.

Thus, the concept of psychopathy is being gradually nibbled away as we learn first about one causal factor and then another, but there are still many individuals who suffer from the disorder in whom no clear-cut precipitating factors can be found at all. The term "Psychopathy" is used very loosely by many people and sometimes it includes men and women who are not truly psychopathic. For example, if a person is brought up in a criminal household his values may well be very different from the average person's and many of his activities are likely to be antisocial. Yet his upbringing may have been normal from the point of view of the parental care he received and he himself may have a normal range of emotions, even if he expresses them somewhat uninhibitedly. In the true sense of the term these people are not psychopaths and should not be described as such.

Psychopathy is a long-term disorder of the personality, so what is the ultimate fate of the condition and the person who suffers from it? The textbooks usually say hopefully that psychopathy tends to improve with age and that, as the individual reaches his twenties and thirties, his emotions and attitudes mature and his behaviour becomes more stable. This is probably true of a proportion of patients, but nobody is at all sure about the overall outlook in psychopathy. Quite a few psychopaths become addicted to alcohol or drugs and after a time the psychopathic appearances are submerged by the manifestations of these other conditions. There is a high death rate in young psychopaths due to accidents brought about by their own foolhardiness and inability to see the need for caution, and due to violence because of their frequent involvement in quarrels and fights. Quite a high proportion of psychopaths become long-term prison inmates and others are incarcerated in mental hospitals or institutions for the criminally insane. Those who show psychological instability often develop other forms of psychiatric illness after a time and these may overshadow the personality disorder: quite frequently these patients attempt suicide and many succeed in killing themselves. It is our view that the long-term prospect in this condition is a remarkably poor one, with a high morbidity and mortality rate and with many cases failing to show any marked improvement in their social conduct over a considerable period.

The treatment of psychopathy is an uncertain business. Most of these individuals do not regard themselves as unwell and do not seek treatment for their condition. Mostly they are young and extremely restless and continuity of treatment is very difficult to ensure. Many of the psychopaths who come for psychiatric treatment do so because they have committed some offence and have been found by the authorities to be psychologically abnormal. As a result they arrive at the psychiatric department either with a grudge at being forced to attend or else pleased with themselves because they think they have received a "soft option" to a prison sentence. If they have sufficient sense they give the appearance of co-operation for a time, but very often they are essentially unwilling patients. Even those psychopaths who are genuinely willing to have treatment at first are liable to abandon it on a whim and disappear.

The psychopath is often group-disruptive and he regularly displays a great deal of provocative behaviour which is very disturbing to non-psychopathic patients. It is better, therefore, to treat him in a special unit which caters for his particular disorder. Nowadays this type of unit often functions as a Therapeutic Community in which every aspect of the environment is employed as an aid to treatment. Psychotherapy, and especially group psychotherapy, is widely used and the daily routine is largely a responsibility of the patients themselves. The rationale of this approach is the development of the psychopath's hitherto underdeveloped communal sense, the encouragement to develop responsible attitudes and realistic goals towards which he can begin consistently to work. There is no firm evidence that this form of treatment encourages psychopathy to clear up any more rapidly than it would do of its own accord and it is quite ineffective with the severer forms of the condition. Its greatest use is probably in the inculcation of healthier attitudes in those individuals who are already in the process of maturing. Some authorities would maintain that an authoritarian approach is just as effective in encouraging the appearance of a social conscience and greater responsibility. Of course, in those cases where the psychopathic behaviour is related to brain damage or epilepsy drug treatment may be required, but at the same time supervision will be necessary until the patient is demonstrably more stable. Psychotherapy is often necessary in the maturing psychopath to enable him to cope with new emotions and relationships and to help him to come to terms with a more settled way of life.

We have already sounded a warning to the social worker who will have to deal with psychopaths because it is essential that she should know exactly on what sort of terms she must meet him. Whether she is asked to see him as a client or comes across him as the relative of a patient, he is unlikely to be a very encouraging prospect. So long as it pays him to be pleasant he will be so, but essentially he is difficult and irresponsible and if he does not get his own way he may become unpleasant and even aggressive in his manner. As he is usually good at deceiving people he will naturally try to hoodwink you. Not infrequently he will succeed, but he will succeed less often if you are fully aware of his proclivities. If he does manage to gain some advantage over you it will encourage him to try the ruse again, so it is necessary to make him aware that you are not going to be taken in readily. If he is a patient, show him that you are prepared to offer kindness and help, but on your terms rather than his.

The relatives of a psychopath are often in sore straits because of his wayward behaviour and it is remarkable how frequently they fail to see through him for a very long time. When the social worker is dealing with these non-psychopathic relatives it is her task to help them with the problems that are brought about by the patient's irresponsibility and try to help them adopt a realistic and insightful attitude to his misdeeds. Sometimes the situation is quite hopeless and it is obvious that the patient has no intention of changing his behaviour. In these circumstances the realities of the problem should be discussed with the relatives, and the social worker should also discuss them carefully with the psychiatrist. If it is considered that the psychopath cannot be reformed, then there is no need for the social worker to make heroic efforts to save the domestic situation for his benefit. She may encourage the relatives to talk out their anxieties so that they can more readily make a personal decision, but she must never be tempted to give outright advice to someone to break up a marriage because the spouse is psychopathic, unless under the most exceptional circumstances and then only after consultation. Advice of this sort is potentially actionable but, more important than this, it is vital that such an important decision should be made by the person without any form of coercion. Unfortunately, the psychopath frequently has a disturbing effect on the people with whom he comes in close contact and he produces disruptive effects on society generally. There is an increasing demand on the social worker to try to remove or prevent the problems which result from this behaviour. Unlike many of the referrals which come her way, the social worker cannot always count on getting as much support from her psychiatric colleagues as she would like because of the intractable nature of this condition. We feel, therefore, that it is worth repeating our warning of the dangers of becoming over-involved in the social problems of the psychopath by acceding to his demands too quickly or by being too optimistic about the prognosis. There is of course a danger that the term "psychopath" will be used to include all the patients or clients whose behaviour we cannot tolerate or alleviate and the temptation to do this must also be avoided.

Psychosexual Disorders

The subject of sex is still bound up to a very great extent in myth and taboo and it is only in recent years that any really factual material on the physical, psychological and social aspects of the subject have become available. Of its nature it is a highly emotive topic and it will continue to be extremely controversial for a long time yet. Present-day society is utterly confused in its approach to sex and it is still trying to reconcile age-old moral views with the permissiveness of modern behaviour. Data are accruing to suggest that many ideas which have hitherto been considered to be common sense are in fact quite erroneous. In this bewildering situation, psychiatry is faced with the problem of trying to differentiate between the normal and the abnormal in sexual matters and of attempting to devise methods of treatment which will cure deviations from normality.

Everyday observation would lead us to believe that there are two sexes which are physically and psychologically distinct but which are biologically complementary for the purpose of mating and procreation. In general terms this is true in that there are genetic differences which determine the obvious physical distinctions between the sexes. However, a variety of pathological influences can act on the developing foetus and these may so alter the physical appearance that a member of one sex can come to appear almost indistinguishable from a member of the opposite sex. Thus, on the physical level, it has become obvious that there is no absolute dividing line between the sexes. Rather surprisingly, it would appear that the very young infant is capable of being influenced to function psychologically as a member of its own or the opposite sex. When a child is born, its physical appearance causes it to be assigned to the appropriate sexual category and thereafter it is the attitude of its parents and other adults which will largely determine its psychosexual orientation. If it happens that the child is genetically male but, by an accident of development, has assumed a female appearance, it may be raised as a female and have all the appropriate psychological attributes: and vice versa. Even where the genetic sex and the sexual appearance are in agreement, numerous adverse influences can act on the child during the course of psychological development to divert, halt, reverse or even banish psychosexual maturation. The end result is that, on the psychological and emotional planes, no one is completely male or female. We are all a mixture of these attributes, though in the normal man there will be a considerable predominance of male attitudes and, in the normal woman, a preponderance of female attitudes.

When the development of the sexual drive has been adversely affected for some reason, a variety of effects may result. The drive may be reduced in intensity, causing lack of interest in sexual matters with impotence in the man and frigidity in the woman. It may be diverted so that sexual attraction is felt towards a member of the same rather than the opposite sex or it may be altered so that there are abnormalities in the manner in which the person obtains sexual satisfaction (as, for example, when masturbation is preferred to normal coitus). It is now realized that normal people indulge in a very wide range of sexual activities and it would appear that most forms of sexual behaviour can be regarded as acceptable if both partners are happy with them. If some form of behaviour which is regarded as perverted is indulged in to the exclusion of other more acceptable forms, then this may be regarded as abnormal, but even here the decision is often a moral and social, rather than a medical, one.

Sexual activity is part of the mechanism to ensure procreation of the species and in a biological sense it is only behaviour which seriously interferes with procreation which can truly be regarded as abnormal. However, it is almost impossible to extricate this aspect from the tangle of social and moral beliefs which determine our opinions on what is right and wrong in sex. Homosexuality is generally considered morally wrong, yet it appears to occur in every human society and it also presents a biological paradox in that it effectively reduces fertility by preventing normal sexual intercourse. To add to the paradox, it is known that homosexual forms of behaviour are fairly common in many lower animals: this may be due to absence of partners of the opposite sex during the mating season, but it also occurs as habitual behaviour in certain individuals. One possible explanation of such anti-reproductive behaviour may be that it ensures that unsuitable members of the species do not pass on their undesirable characteristics to subsequent generations. Whatever its rationale, it is certainly true that a sexual "abnormality" like homosexuality is common and will keep on cropping up in one generation after another.

At the present time we can say that certain forms of sexual behaviour are socially unacceptable and perhaps even biologically disadvantageous, but we still remain relatively ignorant of the actual patterns of sexual mores within our own species. When an individual complains of a sexual disorder one has first of all to decide whether it really is a disorder or whether the individual's ignorance has led him to think that it is. Thereafter, it is necessary to sort out the actual abnormality from this reaction to it. For example, many homosexuals regard their sexual preferences as perfectly normal but are aware of society's disapproval: so they hide their predilections and the stress of this may make them tense and depressed. Again, a man may have a rather weak libido but be otherwise sexually normal and he may complain of anxiety because he imagines he is not satisfying his wife or he is not as potent as other men. As we shall show, it is necessary to make an accurate assessment of his complaint in order to decide whether we tackle the sexual deviation itself or the psychological symptoms which are secondary to it. There is a very great need for accurate and sensible sex education in the general population, but fortunately it is not our responsibility to tackle the vexed question of who should provide this.

Masturbation

Erotic self-stimulation used to be regarded as a sign of moral degeneracy and it was thought that it produced all sorts of serious physical and mental disorders. In fact, the great majority of males practise this habit to a greater or lesser extent during adolescence and some may continue to do so thereafter. A fairly high proportion of women have also indulged in masturbation at some time or another. In itself it appears to be a fairly harmless activity which does not cause any noticeable damage, but it often generates a great deal of guilt and shame in adolescents, who regard it as a sign of profound weakness that they cannot resist the habit. Most often masturbation is used as a means of obtaining some form of sexual gratification when other forms are not attainable. It may become undesirable when it comes to be employed as a means of reducing non-sexual forms of tension. When this happens it may come to have an almost compulsive quality and may become partly divorced from sexual fantasy. Masturbation is not a cause of mental illness, but excessive masturbation is sometimes evidence that the individual is tending to retreat from reality instead of maturing towards normal social and sexual relationships.

Adolescents who are anxious about masturbation can best be helped if they are given the opportunity to discuss the matter with someone they can trust, who certainly need not be a psychiatrist. Simple reassurance is often all that is necessary, but they should usually be encouraged to widen their interests and they may require help if they are socially gauche. Ultimately the best remedy is being able to enter into a stable sexual relationship, but of course this must necessarily be a long-term prospect for many adolescents. It is only in the minority of cases in which masturbation is a sign of some deeper psychological disturbance that actual treatment is necessary.

Impotence

Potency is the ability of a male to have normal sexual intercourse, and this is not synonymous with fertility as many infertile men can still enjoy satisfactory sexual relations. In order that coitus may occur the male has to experience sexual desire which should lead to erection of the penis. Thereafter, the female vagina is entered and following a variable period of time the man experiences orgasm which is usually accompanied by ejaculation. If he is unable to go through this process for any reason, so that normal coitus cannot take place, he is considered to be impotent. Impotence can arise in a variety of ways. In the first place there may be a lack of sexual desire, which, in some people, may be a permanent state due to some failure of psychological development and in others is a temporary state due to exhaustion, depressive illness, anxiety or an unsatisfactory relationship with the sexual partner. The impotence may be relative and in some men is due to a strong element of latent homosexuality which effectively makes women sexually unattractive to them: in others it is due to an inability to feel sexual attraction towards a particular woman, though their relations with other women may be normal. The lack of potency is not always complete and, for example, some men suffer from Premature Ejaculation, a condition in which the male orgasm occurs much too soon and as a result the woman is unable to reach her climax.

Whatever form the impotence takes, the individual is usually worried and extremely embarrassed by his disability and a long period may elapse before he seeks help. When he does request medical advice it is always necessary to exclude the possibility that the impotence is caused by some form of physical disease, though in fact this is a relatively uncommon cause. It is also necessary to ascertain whether there is any notable degree of psychiatric illness present which could be causing the failure of sexual powers. With the patient's permission the problem may be discussed with his wife and it is often the social worker who is required to go very tactfully into the details of the situation, assessing the wife's attitudes and trying to discover any factors which could have initiated or perpetuated the condition. Sometimes it is found that the difficulty is due to ignorance of sexual matters on the part of one or both partners and simple discussion and explanation is all that is required. However, where definite psychosexual problems exist, the husband may need some form of psychotherapy and in some cases the wife too may require treatment. Even if she does not warrant formal therapy, it is often helpful if the social worker arranges to see the wife at regular intervals to provide sympathetic encouragement. In some cases, anxiety is the main problem and here the use of mild tranquillizing drugs is often indicated. Recently there has been some success in the treatment of premature ejaculation with one particular tranquillizer whose effect on this condition seems fairly specific.

Frigidity

This is the condition in which a woman consistently fails to achieve sexual satisfaction during coitus. It is relatively common and a great many women are even unaware that they are missing a significant experience because they have never had an orgasm at any time. There are innumerable degrees of frigidity and the complete form is often associated with marked psychosexual immaturity. Many frigid women can still have sexual intercourse though they get no enjoyment from it, but in extreme forms of the condition the individual becomes so tense when penetration is attempted that coitus is quite impossible. In the lesser degrees of frigidity, there may be a variety of reasons for failing to experience orgasm. Sometimes it is due to clumsiness or inadequate sexual technique on the part of the man, at other times to fear of pregnancy, to lack of privacy or, in certain cases, to unconscious lesbian tendencies. It may also be due to depression, and since this is common after childbirth a period of relative frigidity is not infrequent at this time.

Since frigidity is a less obvious condition than impotence it may not be complained of at all, or it may on occasion be the husband who complains of his wife's unresponsiveness. When the condition comes to notice, it is again necessary to carry out a full physical and psychological examination to exclude any specific illnesses which might be causing it. If it is obvious that the cause is emotional it is usually wise to arrange for both wife and husband to be interviewed, and sometimes the psychiatrist who finds himself dealing with an excessively reticent and embarrassed wife may find it advantageous to ask a female social worker to discuss the sexual problem with the wife while he interviews the husband. In the simplest cases, discussion and advice on sexual matters may be sufficient. In others, the wife and possibly the husband may require psychotherapy to deal with deep-seated fears, and drugs to allay anxiety. There are occasions when it transpires that the wife's "frigidity" is really a failure of satisfaction due to the husband's premature ejaculation, and then it is the husband who has to have the treatment.

Male Homosexuality

Males and females go through a stage in early adolescence when their sexual emotions are beginning to increase in intensity but have not become permanently orientated. This is often a period of "crushes", sometimes on members of the same sex, and in a proportion of cases a certain amount of mild sexual behaviour may occur within groups of boys or girls. Normally this stage is passed fairly quickly and the interest becomes almost completely heterosexual, but in certain individuals a partial or complete arrest of psychosexual development occurs for some reason at this time. Sometimes this simply results in a mild degree of latent homosexual emotion, but in extreme cases there is exclusively homosexual orientation. Between the heterosexual and the homosexual male is a complete spectrum of sexual orientation and in some circumstances (as when men are confined together in prison) apparently normal males will seek sexual gratification in homosexual behaviour. When the circumstances return to normal and women become available, the homosexual acts cease.

Male homosexuality is a fairly common condition. Its actual frequency is unknown but it has been estimated that perhaps 5 per cent of adult males are actively practising homosexuals. The great majority of them remain unrecognized and their everyday behaviour does not distinguish them from other men. Many have sufficient heterosexual capacity to get married and even have families. The effeminate "pansy" is the exception rather than the rule, as is the homosexual who makes himself offensive by importuning other males or flaunting his abnormality, and such people are usually suffering from a well-marked degree of personality disorder as well as the sexual problem.

Homosexuality is a form of behaviour found in every human society and it is usually frowned upon, though in a few societies (as, for example, Classical Greece) it has been tolerated and even commended. When toleration is practised the condition appears to become commoner, but this is probably largely due to the number of covert homosexuals who are then willing to declare themselves. This process appears to be occurring in Western society today, though till recently homosexuals were a persecuted minority, liable to blackmail if an unscrupulous individual discovered that they were practising their deviant behaviour or to punishment if they were discovered by the authorities. Unfortunately, at the present time there is something of a tendency for growing tolerance to be interpreted as licence and for some homosexual individuals to obtain undue publicity for themselves. There are probably fairly large numbers of impressionable adolescents who have problems of sexual identity who could be influenced into becoming overtly homosexual if sufficient pressure were applied. Since it is generally believed that homosexuality is a result of a failure of complete development in one aspect of an individual's emotional field, it seems to us wrong to glamorize or unduly publicize the condition as desirable. In our view, this attitude of non-commendation is compatible with an attitude of toleration towards the already confirmed homosexual whose abnormality is not of his own making.

The causes of homosexuality remain to a great extent obscure. The condition is not related to hermaphroditism where the individual actually possesses physical characteristics of both sexes, and it does not appear to be produced by abnormalities of the sex chromosomes or by any other chromosomal disorders. Most male homosexuals appear perfectly normal in constitution and physique and there is usually no evidence of any hormone disturbance. The most strongly homosexual individuals frequently display abnormal traits at a relatively early stage of life, whereas the youth who has an uncertain sexual orientation may become abnormal as the result of seduction by another male during adolescence.

While the deviation usually becomes obvious at puberty, it is probable that the basis of the condition has been formed much earlier in life. Numerous psychological theories have been proposed to account for the development of the predisposition. Most of these claim that there has been a disturbed relationship with the parents. In some cases the individual may reject the image of his father because he was too passive a parent or else he was consistently hostile, and in these circumstances the patient will over-identify with mother. In other cases there may be marked hostility towards mother and, as a result, hostility towards women in general or else mother may be so over-possessive that the individual's developing personality is swamped and he is unable to identify with his male peers. If the child reaches the Oedipal stage with severe emotional disturbances as a result of such conflicts he may not identify adequately with father and thereafter his male role will be uncertain. No one hypothesis has provided an answer to the origin of homosexuality and the reason for its considerable frequency, but there is certainly general agreement that there is an underlying failure of emotional development. In a few cases, homosexual behaviour appears suddenly in someone who has previously been normal: in a young person this is occasionally due to the onset of schizophrenia and in an elderly person to the appearance of a dementing condition.

The exclusively homosexual individual regards sexual relationships with women as repugnant, in fact just as distasteful as the way in which the normal male would regard homosexual acts. He often regards his state as being the norm and unless his deviation makes him feel anxious or guilty he may not suffer at all as a result of it. Nevertheless, it is difficult for homosexuals to form stable relationships with other males. A normal man will indignantly reject any sexual advances, and even if the homosexual does find a willing partner, society frowns on all-male households and so he often has to have recourse to casual encounters in order to gratify his sexual emotions. Even in an atmosphere of growing tolerance he may not dare to reveal his true inclinations. Some homosexuals may be able to get into a type of work or way of life where their deviation is more acceptable—for example, dress-making or some branches of the entertainments industry—but most of them conceal the disorder from other people. This often gives rise to a good deal of tension, especially if they are also maintaining the pretence of a normal marriage. As a result the less stable individual may break down and develop some form of psychiatric illness, or else he may over-compensate by flaunting his abnormality or by committing some form of public indecency.

A homosexual may be referred for treatment because his deviation is making him unhappy, because on an intellectual level he regards it as wrong, or because he has got into trouble with the authorities and has been ordered to seek help. In deciding on his suitability for treatment it is necessary to assess his reasons for attending and the degree of motivation he possesses. If it is found that he basically wishes to remain as he is it is usually impossible to re-orientate his sexual emotions, though it may be possible to help him with any secondary psychological problems. If he suffers from a marked degree of personality disturbance in addition to his homosexuality (and this is true of a considerable proportion of the group who have been in trouble with the authorities) it is very unlikely that he will persist with any treatment. The man who is exclusively homosexual is not likely to respond to therapy, but if he has *some* degree of heterosexual interest the chances of helping him are greatly improved.

Treatment has traditionally been by psychotherapy, and the treatment has aimed at allowing the patient to work through the emotional disturbances which have delayed emotional maturity. It has also attempted to provide him with a stronger male image with which to identify. Although optimistic claims have sometimes been made by individual practitioners the over-all success rate is not high with psychotherapeutic methods of treatment. At present, encouraging reports are emerging about the beneficial effects of behaviour therapy. In this form of treatment the patient is taught, by means of unpleasant associative stimuli, to dislike homosexuality, and at the same time he is persuaded to think of heterosexual matters in a pleasurable way. By repeatedly applying these conditions, his sexual orientation may be radically altered. There is no doubt that these changes occur, but behaviour therapy is still in the experimental stage and it is necessary not to be over-optimistic about its effects. All the same, it does seem as though it offers a hope of cure in many cases without the necessity for going through the lengthy, costly and often unsuccessful process of psychotherapy.

Moral admonition and common-sense advice have little to offer in the treatment of homosexuality. Sometimes they drive it out of sight but the resultant stress on the personality may cause profound harm. Many homosexuals have married in a desperate hope that this will cure them, but often this leads to disastrous results for both them and their wives. If the man is fortunate and treatment is helping him, he must learn to adapt to a whole new way of life and to do this he may require a good deal of support and sympathetic help. Homosexuals tend to form their own exclusive social groups and it may be difficult to break away from these and establish links with normal society. In offering help the social worker must be friendly and non-moralistic, but at the same time she can still strive in most cases to present the view that normal standards of sexual behaviour are a desirable goal for the individual to attain. Where the personality is a severely disordered one the problems are considerably greater, and we have given earlier in this chapter some consideration to the ways in which they should be tackled.

Lesbianism

Female homosexuality is possibly as common as the male variety, but its presence in the community is much less obvious. Lesbian practices are not punishable in this country unless they constitute a public nuisance and this rarely happens. The general public is very tolerant of certain aspects of female behaviour which it would find quite unacceptable in men, such as kissing, embracing and walking hand-in-hand. Most of the women who behave like this are perfectly normal, but it does mean that no one is very disturbed if two women show a good deal of physical affection towards each other, even in public. As well as this, most populations contain a surplus of women and so all-female households are common enough not to be commented upon. (With the possibility of a surplus of males rapidly approaching, it will be interesting to see whether this public attitude will change.) Most lesbian women are content to keep their homosexual inclinations hidden from general view and it is only the most psychopathic among them who make a show of their abnormality, so to a great extent other people remain ignorant of the condition.

This being so, it is not very common for women to seek treatment for their lesbianism. It is more likely to be found incidentally as one factor in a wider disorder of the personality and it will usually be treated within this context.

Other Forms of Sexual Disorder

Almost every aspect of human sexuality is capable of being perverted in some way and the result is a variety of sexual deviations, all of them morbidly fascinating but not necessarily of great significance to the social worker. They mostly represent some failure of adequate emotional development, though in some instances (as, for example, when sexual pleasure arises from inflicting or receiving pain) there appears to be sexual investment of essentially non-sexual forms of behaviour. The majority of sexual deviations exist quietly in the general population and do not come to psychiatric attention either because the individual can contain his abnormal feelings or has been able to obtain expression for them in a relatively harmless way (perhaps by finding a sexual partner who is prepared to co-operate in his fantasies). Sometimes the deviation is associated with marked compulsive symptoms so that the person has an irresistible desire to gratify his sexual urges even when there is danger in doing this. The dangerous element may even be part of the pleasure, but this type of behaviour frequently lands the individual in trouble. In others, who are nearly always males, sexual abnormalities are combined with aggressiveness and psychopathic traits and this may result in crimes of sexual violence and even murder. Women not uncommonly indulge in perverted practices but to a lesser extent than men and usually more discreetly, though many prostitutes might be regarded as sexually perverse since they are prepared to co-operate in almost any form of obscene behaviour.

We have already described the commonest sexual disorders, and we shall now mention very briefly several of the more important remaining conditions.

1. *Sado-masochism* is a condition in which sexual enjoyment is obtained from the infliction of physical or mental pain (sadism) or from the receiving of hurt and humiliation (masochism). Though not invariably so, men more often tend to be sadistic and women masochistic. Minor forms of such behaviour are very common (for example, lovers' bites) and cannot be regarded as abnormal, but severe sadistic tendencies may sometimes lead to the most abominable acts of cruelty and crime.

2. *Voyeurism* is a form of behaviour in which the individual obtains sexual pleasure from "Peeping Tom" activities. In some cases the sexual stimulant is simply the sight of nakedness or sexual activity in others, but there is often pleasure in the actual peeping and in the possibility of being caught in the act.

3. *Exhibitionism*, in which a man exposes his genitalia to a woman or to a child in the mistaken hope that this will arouse sexual interest. Naturally it rarely does, but quite often the fear or disgust the action produces in the other person is sufficient to lead to orgasm. Indecent exposure often occurs in inadequate, excessively shy men who are sometimes of below-average intelligence and they show a marked tendency to repeat the offence despite punishment.

4. *Transvestism* is characterized by the individual's receiving sexual stimulation from dressing in the clothes of the opposite sex. Again it is largely restricted to men and it is not invariably associated with homosexuality. Many transvestites dress in elaborate and even bizarre female costume and yet their fantasies and behaviour are not infrequently heterosexual.

5. *Trans-sexualism* is a relatively uncommon condition but often gains a great deal of prurient publicity when some individual

undergoes a "sex change" operation. The trans-sexualist (usually a male, but occasionally a woman) is convinced against all reason that he is actually a member of the opposite sex. He claims to have the mind of a woman and insists that it is accidental that he is physically male. He may even deny his maleness and claim that he is menstruating or has become pregnant. Some trans-sexualists are extremely importunate and manage to persuade surgeons to perform plastic operations and give hormone therapy to provide some semblance of reality to their fantasies. To the outsider the results often appear ludicrous, but the individual is sometimes much happier following the operation. In this country such a procedure is regarded as immoral, but conventional psychiatric treatment is often unavailing and many trans-sexualists go on being unhappy, haunted people who can never attain a normal sexual image.

In all the sexual abnormalities the patient may be referred for treatment because he is unhappy with his condition or because he has created some form of public nuisance. In each case the psychiatrist must assess the strength of his motivation to obtain cure and he must decide whether the disorder is relatively discrete or whether it is an expression of a highly disturbed personality. Sometimes the abnormal sexuality is prominent because it is being used by the personality in an attempt to reduce general tension symptoms and in this instance treatment would be directed more towards the reduction of the tension. At other times the deviation is present in its own right, and where a real desire for cure is present the most appropriate form of treatment, whether it be behaviour therapy, psychotherapy or other, must be chosen. When the social worker is involved in the case she often has to deal with the relatives and it is evident that a great deal of tact and discretion is necessary. The family is often horrified that a member should have got into disgrace or have transgressed the conventional moral code and they may have to be given a great deal of help and support before they can come to appreciate the individual's problems.

People with severe sexual abnormalities are particularly liable to land in trouble. When an individual has sought help before he has openly broken any law the psychiatrist and the social worker will, of course, respect his confidence and treat his condition as an illness and not as an offence. Only rarely is it necessary to break this confidence and then only under the most exceptional circumstances, as when there is a strong likelihood that the patient will commit a crime of sexual violence. In such a situation the decision to break confidence must be the psychiatrist's alone. If a patient has already committed a crime and been punished for this it is normally our duty to work within the context of the law and to treat the condition during or after the course of the penalty. In some cases we are justified in making attempts to have the punishment alleviated if the sexual abnormality has been sufficiently severe to interfere with the individual's restraint and judgement, but it is not usually part of our work to help someone avoid the consequences of having committed a public offence. Fortunately, the law is nowadays adopting a much more flexible attitude towards the whole problem of sexual deviations.

CHAPTER 7

Alcoholism and Drug Addiction

Alcoholism

The problem of alcoholism is a very large and complex one in modern societies. Apart from Muslim countries, most communities condone and even encourage the drinking of alcohol, and where this is so inevitably a certain proportion of the population will become addicted to it. Patterns of drinking vary from place to place and this results in considerable variation in the frequency with which public drunkenness occurs and also in the frequency of alcoholism and its serious mental and physical effects.

It is important not to confuse drunkenness with alcoholism. Anyone who drinks alcohol may on occasion become inebriated and some people frequently do so. Some heavy drinkers are simply following the prevailing cultural pattern of their environment, where it is the norm to go out with one's friends on certain evenings in the week in order to get hopelessly drunk. Other people drink because they have severe problems, either temporary or permanent, and they have found that alcohol can make life more tolerable for the time being. Heavy drinking of these sorts does not necessarily amount to alcoholism because most of the individuals can stop drinking when they want to, or have to, and they suffer no particular ill-effects when this happens. But amongst the heavy drinkers there are people who can no longer stop when they want to. They have lost control of their drinking and if they take just one alcoholic drink they have an overwhelming desire to take more and more until they are utterly inebriated. When this stage has been reached the person has become an Alcohol Addict. After a period of time, constant abuse of alcohol begins to produce severe physical and mental effects (which we shall mention later) and if the alcoholic stops drinking he may develop severe withdrawal symptoms. By this time he is a very sick man indeed and his condition is now known as Chronic Alcoholism.

In this country, alcohol addiction is a very serious problem and it has been estimated that there are more than a quarter of a million alcoholics in Britain. Perhaps one in four of these show evidence of some damage to their health as a result of excessive drinking. Many of these people do not come to medical or psychiatric attention and some of them would be highly indignant if it were suggested that they were psychologically ill or even that they drank too much. It is indeed possible that, if an alcoholic has a moderately stable personality, if his home and family do not disintegrate and if he takes a regular and adequate diet, he may never break down into a psychiatric illness, but he is still in a sense a very sick man. He is often known to his acquaintances as someone to whom drink is a problem and who is frequently drunk, but he may remain surprisingly healthy in other ways and his behaviour may be tolerated indefinitely by his social circle.

On the other hand, if the alcoholic already has a seriously disturbed personality before he becomes addicted (as is not uncommonly the case), and if he becomes neglected and destitute, causes his family to break up and fails to take a reasonable diet, his physical health may become seriously impaired and he may eventually develop evidence of brain damage. As his mental capacities deteriorate and his judgement becomes affected his drinking is likely to become even heavier and his habits more irregular. Sooner or later he may well land in hospital, either to have treatment for a physical complication of his alcoholism such as cirrhosis of the liver or to have treatment for psychiatric symptoms.

Alcoholism is found predominantly in men, though nowadays the number of female alcoholics is increasing. Until fairly recently there were strong public sanctions against drinking by women and female drunkenness is even yet considered widely to be abhorrent, especially by other women. However, these taboos are much less stringent than they were, so more women drink to excess and a number become alcoholics in the course of time.

Apart from this sex difference there are cultural and social differences in the patterns of drinking, drunkenness and alcoholism. For example, in Scotland it is customary for large amounts of spirits to be consumed and the pattern of drinking is one in which considerable quantities are drunk in a short time. Therefore there is a high incidence of drunkenness and alcoholism occurs more commonly than in England. In the latter country, beer is the predominant form of alcoholic drink and there is less emphasis on rapid consumption, so drunkenness is less prevalent and alcoholism rather less common. In France, public drunkenness is the exception but alcoholism is very common because the steady consumption of large quantities of wine is the rule, and there is a high frequency of the serious physical complications of excessive drinking such as liver damage. Thus the prevalence of alcoholism and the ways in which it presents are dependent on a variety of social factors.

The Aetiology of Alcoholism

Many people are psychologically dependent on alcohol to the extent that they can only be relaxed in company when they have taken a few drinks, but if drink is forbidden for some reason they can usually do without it, albeit with an ill grace. The alcoholic is different. He has passed through some mysterious barrier which relatively few people reach and he has become physically as well as mentally dependent on alcohol which is no longer a beverage to him, but a drug. It has often been postulated that alcoholics undergo some biochemical alteration because they come to react differently to the substance from normal. Many alcoholics can consume enormous quantities of alcohol without appearing to become inebriated, but some, especially in the advanced stages of the condition, become unduly sensitive to its effects and develop intoxication after drinking a small amount. It has even been suggested that alcoholics start life by being biochemically different from other people. This seems a possibility since a great many people drink but it is always only a small proportion who go on to develop addiction.

The rate at which a person becomes an alcoholic varies from one individual to another. Most of the alcoholics who come to medical attention are in their forties or fifties and the condition has often been present for ten or more years before that. A history is often obtained of excessive drinking beginning in the early twenties or even earlier. In contrast to this, some people become addicted to alcohol very rapidly and they may become typical alcoholics within two or three years of starting to drink excessively. The reasons for this seem to be partly constitutional and partly environmental. In these rapid onset cases the basic personality is often a disturbed one, but sometimes there is a history of, for instance, head injury with subsequent personality change and uncontrolled drinking.

The individual who is brought up in a cultural setting where heavy and frequent drinking is the norm is obviously quite likely to become a heavy drinker himself and thus his chances of becoming an alcoholic are increased. It is well known that occupation also has some effect and those people who work in the drink trade are especially at risk, as are those business men and commercial travellers who transact a good deal of their trade over a drink. Men who are involved in physically taxing occupations with a great deal of fluid-loss due to sweating (such as furnacemen or stevedores) often replace fluid by consuming very large amounts of beer. However, in every case the question of the influence of the individual's occupation must be considered with a certain amount of reservation since some people undoubtedly select particular types of work with a view to the amount of alcohol they can consume as part of the job.

In some instances alcoholism appears to arise from another psychiatric condition such as chronic anxiety or depression, when the individual has initially taken to drink to lessen his symptoms and has gradually become dependent upon it. This is probably a fairly uncommon reason for becoming an alcoholic and it is probably the basic personality which is more important in deciding who shall become addicted. Many alcoholics have evidence of considerable psychological problems prior to their developing a dependence on drink. Sometimes the personality disorder consists of general feelings of inadequacy which are alleviated when the person has had a few drinks and gradually this habit becomes more compelling. In other patients the personality abnormalities are a good deal more severe and psychopaths are particularly prone to take to drink. In psychoanalytic theory it is postulated that the alcoholic is someone whose emotional development has been halted at the oral narcissistic stage and who has sexual problems which largely stem from unresolved Oedipal conflicts. Although he may be effectively fairly heterosexual it is suggested that he is latently homosexual as a result of these conflicts. Therefore he is likely to be more at ease in the company of other men and the atmosphere of a public bar is especially congenial to him because it is predominantly masculine and the most important activity, drinking, can assuage his oral needs and also reduce his anxieties. Certainly some alcoholics do have sexual problems and Freud's theory may be true for a certain proportion of them, but it does not explain the aetiology of alcoholism in general.

The Alcoholic's Progress

This, like the Rake's Progress, is usually a story of advancing psychological deterioration and social degradation. In most cases the individual begins by drinking to excess for a considerable time, usually in a social setting. After a time he finds that he cannot drink in moderation any longer and whenever he takes alcohol he inevitably goes on to become inebriated. This often leads to feelings of shame and he may begin to drink alone, usually with the intention of getting drunk. Thereafter he starts to drink at all hours of the day, even to the extent of eventually having to have a drink to start the day. By this time he has often switched from drinking beer to drinking wine or spirits in order to get a greater effect more quickly. In order to afford this he may have to do without food and this means that most of his caloric intake is obtained from alcohol. Since alcohol contains few vitamins he may eventually develop a vitamin-deficiency state, leading to severe physical and mental symptoms. At this stage he is rarely completely sober for any length of time and his work suffers accordingly, so he probably starts to lose jobs. If he does not have enough money for drink he cadges or even steals and his sense of morality becomes subservient to the need for alcohol. He may still be able to keep up some sort of façade of bonhomie when he is with his drinking friends (if he has any), but at home he is usually irritable and difficult towards his wife and family who are often by now semi-destitute. On occasion he may become violent while in his cups.

As the condition progresses the alcoholic begins to have "black-outs", varying periods of time for which he has no recollection afterwards and which are usually related to severe bouts of drinking. Physical ailments secondary to the alcoholism begin to appear, including chronic stomach disorders, liver disease and chronic bronchitis. Mental changes also become prominent, so that he is facile and utterly lacking in insight. If he tries to stop drinking or simply runs out of money to buy a drink, he may well develop delirium tremens (see below). In the most severe cases of chronic alcoholism there may be hallucinations and well-marked delusions, and in some instances severe dementia occurs as a result of brain damage. (This brain damage is not due to the directly poisonous effect of the alcohol itself but to the lack of vitamins, especially those of the B group, which results from the inadequate food-intake.) Some individuals become utterly destitute and degraded and stop drinking ethyl alcohol, the normal basis for alcoholic drinks, drinking instead methyl alcohol, which is a severe poison. In all severe alcoholics the physical constitution becomes undermined and constant self-neglect can lead to the development of illnesses like pneumonia which may, in some cases, cause death.

The Complications of Alcoholism

Taken in sufficient quantities alcohol is a poison which can produce coma and even death, but most alcoholics build up such an enormous tolerance that they rarely die of acute alcoholic intoxication.

Delirium tremens. After years of excessive drinking an individual may start to have attacks of delirium tremens (often known as D.T.s). This condition usually occurs when the alcoholic suddenly stops drinking for some reason or it may be precipitated by an acute illness, particularly one associated with fever. An attack often begins gradually, starting with feelings of anxiety and restlessness and continuing with tremulousness and severe malaise. The patient is nauseated by food, so he stops eating. The anxiety feelings progress to sensations of dread and panic and hallucinations may appear. These are usually visual and consist of little beasts and crawling creatures rather than the legendary pink elephant. Delirium with confusion and disorientation supervenes and the patient is obviously seriously ill, with profuse sweating and marked tremor. Insomnia is very severe and may continue throughout the attack, which can last up to a week. Sometimes convulsions occur and it is not unknown for a patient to die during a severe attack of delirium tremens. The condition has to be treated as an acute medical emergency, but with adequate treatment the patient should make a rapid recovery.

Korsakow's state. This is a form of organic psychosis which sometimes arises in a very severe chronic alcoholic. It is characterized by almost complete disorientation for time and place and by an almost total inability to remember recent events, though distant memories are often well retained. Thus the individual may recognize someone he has not met for thirty years but will be quite unable to remember the person whom he saw just a minute or two previously. He often confabulates (that is, he invents fictitious but sometimes probable-sounding details) to cover up his memory disorder, but this does not betoken any insight into his disabilities and he appears bland and euphoric, quite content to lead an aimless, vegetable-like existence. Recovery from a Korsakow state is comparatively rare and the patient usually remains a long-term hospital inmate. Further dementia may occur, resulting in certain neurological abnormalities along with the mental symptoms, and this later stage is known as Wernicke's encephalopathy.

Alcoholic hallucinosis. This is an illness which occurs in some very heavy drinkers. It may start fairly suddenly with the development of delusions or even auditory hallucinations. The individual becomes convinced that other people are talking about him or plotting against him and he often complains that there is an unreal quality about his surroundings. All of this may clear up fairly quickly but sometimes it progresses either to a dementia or to an apparently typical paranoid schizophrenia. In the latter instance, if he is married the patient quite frequently has the delusion that his wife is being unfaithful to him. Alcoholism often leads to impotence and the man misinterprets his inability to satisfy his wife as evidence that she has become sexually insatiable. Thereafter he jumps to the mistaken conclusion that she must be trying to seek satisfaction for her appetites elsewhere. This may lead to violence towards her and occasionally he may commit murder in a frenzy of jealousy.

Pathological intoxication. This is a condition in which the individual becomes confused and apparently intoxicated after consuming small amounts of alcohol and sometimes he may go utterly berserk after one or two drinks. Sometimes this is related to psychopathy, but most often it is an indication that a form of epilepsy is present.

Dipsomania. This is a fairly rare disorder in which a person has periodic severe drinking bouts for which he has no subsequent recollection, while between bouts he is a moderate drinker or even a teetotaller. The condition usually occurs in certain psychopaths who develop periodic tension states and occasionally in individuals who have intermittent attacks of severe depression: in either case the excessive drinking appears to have the effect of relieving the disturbed mood state.

Alcoholism in women. While alcoholism is still predominantly a disease of men, it is becoming decidedly commoner in women. Since the social sanctions against heavy drinking in women are still quite severe, it is usually a woman with a pretty disturbed personality who defies custom to become a chronic alcoholic. Much of her drinking tends to be done at home and this leads to innumerable domestic quarrels. The rate of marriage breakdown in female alcoholics is very high. In general, their response to treatment is extremely poor.

Treatment of Alcoholism

We have been describing what happens to the severe alcoholic, but of course there are many alcoholics whose illness does not progress nearly so far. However, the patients who are referred for psychiatric treatment are often physically debilitated, have undergone a good deal of social degradation and are suffering from severe mental symptoms. Their family life has often been destroyed and in many cases they are leading a hand-to-mouth existence. In the first instance treatment must always be directed at the improvement of the individual's physical condition and the cure of delirium tremens if this is present. The alcoholic should be admitted to hospital, preferably to a psychiatric department which deals specifically with the problems of alcoholism. Total abstinence is insisted upon from the beginning and if the patient is restless or disturbed as a result of withdrawal of the alcohol he will receive adequate sedation for the time being. Any physical conditions are treated and he is encouraged to start eating heartily again. Only after the immediate crisis is over can the psychiatrist assess the patient's suitability or otherwise for treatment.

Quite a few alcoholics become over-confident and even arrogant as soon as they begin to feel better and if this happens it indicates a lack of insight which bodes ill for the success of treatment. Unless an alcoholic can admit that the condition has utterly defeated him and that he needs help, he will rarely persist in therapy. To help him, the psychiatrist must enlist his full co-operation and must make it seem worth while for him to regain his self-esteem. If the patient's underlying personality is even moderately stable he may find reserves within himself to respond to treatment, but where the personality is markedly abnormal the possibility of success is greatly reduced. In the cases in which insight can be achieved, individual or group psychotherapy may be employed. In the course of this the patient is encouraged to develop the sense of responsibility which has lain dormant for so long and to attempt to solve his problems realistically instead of resorting to the whisky bottle on the slightest pretext. He must learn to be utterly frank, and if he has lapses he must admit these to the therapist because if he hides them from the latter he will soon re-enter the maze of lies, self-justification and self-deception which have bedevilled him for so long. Unfortunately many patients fail to complete their treatment and the rate of relapse is high, but they should be given every chance to resume if there seems a reasonable hope of improvement.

In a number of alcoholics, treatment of a physical nature may be employed to deal with the addiction, either in combination with psychotherapy or by itself. In aversion therapy an attempt is made to condition the individual to dislike alcohol. This is usually done by giving him alcoholic drinks and at the same time making him violently sick by means of injections of an emetic drug. This procedure is repeated again and again till he comes to associate the idea of alcohol with feelings of nausea and has no wish to drink any. In some patients this can be very effective but the aversion usually wears off within a year or even less and the whole process may have to be repeated again and again. As may be imagined, the patients do not regard it with any great favour because it is an unpleasant form of treatment, but nevertheless there are some cases where it is extremely beneficial and not a few where it can potentiate other forms of therapy. Another method of physical treatment consists of giving the patient a drug in tablet form which he takes once a day and which will produce severe feelings of nausea and discomfort if he consumes any alcohol within the following 24 hours. The principle here is that the patient soon learns that once he has taken the drug he dare not take a drink for a specific period thereafter or else he will be violently sick. Unfortunately this demands considerable co-operation from the patient and if he really wants to drink it is only too easy for him to stop taking his tablets. As well as this the use of the drug requires some care because it can occasionally produce dangerous side-effects.

The aim of any treatment is to enable the individual to return to a useful and reasonably well-organized life. Many alcoholics have not enjoyed such an existence for a considerable length of time and the effort of trying to attain it again is frequently beyond them, so it is easier to return to the bottle for consolation. The individual who finds it impossible to return to a normal life tends to slip further and further downwards, living in doss-houses or sleeping in the hedgerows and intermittently entering mental hospital or prison. He drifts into hospital, regarding it more as a means of obtaining bed and board than treatment, and drifts out again, better fed and clothed but no nearer cure in most cases. It is rarely legally justifiable to keep chronic alcoholics of this type in hospital against their will, so they go on relentlessly abusing their health until eventually it breaks down or they lose their reason completely. In the worst cases these people may become methylated spirit drinkers and when this occurs the possibility of psychiatric rehabilitation is almost hopeless.

The life of the alcoholic revolves around drink: the need for it, the process of obtaining it and the actual drinking of it. If he gives up drinking there is a very large gap in his everyday existence and if he is to remain abstinent something worth while must be substituted. A return to a decent family life with encouragement from relatives and friends may be sufficient for this purpose in a few cases, or religious conversion may provide the answer for some. At the present time the Alcoholics Anonymous organization is probably the most effective means of providing moral support and human companionship for the newly abstinent alcoholic. It also provides an extremely important "first-aid" service for the individual who fears he may lapse or has actually done so. All the members of Alcoholics Anonymous are themselves ex-alcoholics who are pledged to help each other to remain sober and the organization has done a very great deal to aid the rehabilitation of large numbers of alcoholics. It is no criticism of the Association to say that it is unfortunate that its results are usually best in people with relatively stable personalities: the more psychopathic type of alcoholic tends to drift away sooner or later and to relapse seriously.

Social workers are frequently involved in dealing with cases of alcoholism and quite often this occurs outside the sphere of medical practice. There are many alcoholics who have proved resistant to treatment who drift around the community, utterly down and out, and who represent a challenge for compassion rather than therapy.

On the other hand, there are alcoholics who do not reach a psychiatric break-down point but who may be social problems because their family relationships are deteriorating and their children are becoming disturbed, or who break the law by some form of antisocial behaviour due to drunkenness. If such problems do not reach psychiatric attention the social worker employed by a non-medical agency may have a good deal of responsibility for dealing with the serious difficulties which result. In cases where the drinking is uncontrolled and the individual's personal and family life is disintegrating, attempts must be made to have some form of medical treatment instituted. However, it is as well that we should warn the social worker at this point that she will often find it very difficult to persuade a psychiatrist to deal with a broken-down, psychopathic alcoholic, because he knows from experience that the "Skid Row" alcoholic is usually beyond the reach of treatment, though occasionally within the reach of social or religious influences. It is also fairly certain that the psychiatrist will be unwilling to deal with the alcoholic who has been coerced into seeking treatment. The social worker must appreciate that the alcoholic usually has to be utterly demoralized before he can truly be helped, but she must also realize that he has to have some reserves of personality, however small, in order to learn to take some sort of useful place in society again. If a man has proved to be effectively beyond treatment, this fact must be accepted. Do not break your back or your heart trying to reform him. Instead, give him the sort of practical help that he so badly needs, namely food, shelter and recognition as a human being.

The alcoholic who has learned the vital fact that he cannot take even one drink and who has responded well to treatment will often need social support and practical help in addition to what Alcoholics Anonymous has to offer. He may require assistance to find work, advice in order to get his finances straight again, and encouragement when he tries to break down the barrier of antipathy created by his former drunkenness. There may be times when his problems prove too overwhelming and he turns to the bottle for consolation. Afterwards he experiences remorse and despair and this brings the temptation to drink even more. When this happens he needs sympathy and support: he also needs a human being who provides a stable point of reference and who is prepared to act with authority while remaining non-moralistic. Eventually the aim must be to enable the alcoholic to become self-sufficient and to be relatively free of the need for social work support. Often this ideal can only be partially realized and it is certainly a very good thing for the patient to maintain some kind of contact with the social agency and especially with Alcoholics Anonymous.

The social worker is frequently involved with the family as much as with the alcoholic himself. The way in which the alcoholic's household functions usually depends to a great extent on the personality of the wife and whether she can cope with the enormous difficulties that the patient's behaviour engenders. It has often been noted that the wives of alcoholics tend to differ markedly from other women. Either they are able to deal astonishingly well with their problems or else they are excessively meek and passive women who accept blows and hardship without complaint. In some instances the wife, no matter how ill-used, seems almost to obtain satisfaction from the disturbed relationship. Perhaps it gives her the opportunity to be a mother-figure rather than a wife or perhaps her fatalism reflects an excess of masochism. Quite often she appears to be repeating some sort of life-pattern because the alcoholic's wife is frequently the product of an alcoholic household though not herself an alcoholic. However, no matter the reason for her choice of marriage partner, the constant drunkenness, unreliability and frequently destitution with which she is faced gradually wear her down until she may need psychiatric treatment in her own right. Even if she feels anger and disgust towards her husband she usually has to be placatory towards him in order to maintain some degree of stability for herself and the children. The children suffer a great deal too because the predominant emotions in the household are very often fear and uncertainty and these can have a profoundly damaging effect on the developing personality. It is interesting that so many alcoholics have themselves undergone a deprived childhood of this nature.

Part of the treatment of alcoholism must be directed towards an attempt to make the family situation more stable, partly to help the alcoholic but also because the wife and children need respite. If the patient is unco-operative it may prove very difficult to help the family as he may construe any intervention as part of a plot against him. However, every attempt should be made to give aid firstly on the practical level as regards money, food and clothing, and secondly (and perhaps more important) to give moral encouragement and even psychiatric treatment if it is needed. As a last resort, if the family is inevitably going to break up, the social worker may be called on to give advice and assistance in this situation. If, on the other hand, the patient has responded well to treatment, then the family should be encouraged to rally round him so as to make his environment a warm and secure one in order that that he may have a real incentive to remain abstinent.

Drug Addiction

Drugs of various sorts are now part of everyday living and many people cherish the belief that if they are unwell there will be a tablet to cure them whatever the illness. This is certainly a good deal more true than it was twenty or thirty years ago. However, an impression is gaining ground that there are drugs which will help you not only if you are ill, but will be guaranteed to make you relaxed and happy when you are feeling upset, and many people now regard it as their right to demand this type of chemical euphoria. Nowadays a very large proportion of the drugs prescribed in a modern society are for insomnia, anxiety and depression, conditions which sometimes represent true illnesses but which at other times are states of mind or simple reactions to difficult situations. In many instances these complaints would not have been considered worthy of medical attention until comparatively lately. There is no doubt that many of the people who receive drugs for them do indeed require treatment, but equally there is no doubt that far too many individuals have become unnecessarily dependent on drugs which they take for relatively trivial reasons. In present-day Great

Britain, several million adults regularly take sleeping tablets and one estimate has suggested that possibly two million people are habituated to them. Most of these individuals would vehemently deny that they are virtually drug addicts, and it is true that in most cases the dependence is largely psychological. Nevertheless it is a fact that very many people depend on drugs for their night's sleep *every night*. Many others are prescribed tablets when they are disturbed or anxious because it is easier for them to take drugs than to solve the problems which have caused their psychological symptoms. Psychiatrists are being given more and more sophisticated drugs to combat the symptoms of mental illness and they are becoming more skilled in the use of these, but at the same time far too many people are taking these drugs for prolonged periods for unsuitable reasons.

It could be argued that the symptoms of mild drug-dependence are preferable to the symptoms which the drugs are meant to treat, and it could also be argued that if an individual needs to be sedated or stimulated it is better that this be done in a relatively controlled way with drugs than to allow him to use a substance like alcohol which may have so many unpleasant personal and social side-effects. Unfortunately, drugs also have their side-effects, as we shall show, and there is no doubt that at present they are over-available. Many people who regularly take drugs suffer some degree of intoxication from them. For example, a person who takes a barbiturate sleeping tablet every night can often be shown to be mentally sluggish and to have certain mild physical evidences of the drug's presence throughout the following day. The majority suffer no further ill-effects, though it is not uncommon for the drug gradually to lose its effectiveness, whereupon the dose is increased and the side-effects become more noticeable. There are many middle-aged and elderly people who are in a state of drug-induced semi-intoxication more or less permanently. Usually if the drug is stopped there is an initial period of severe insomnia and this makes the patient unwilling to cease from taking it.

The person who has gone beyond the stage of taking drugs for their therapeutic effect and who takes them for their own sake may feel very unwell if he cannot have access to them and he often shows a marked tendency to keep increasing the dose. This dependence is at first to a great extent psychological and at this stage the individual is said to be habituated to the drug. If he goes a stage further he develops an actual physical dependence on the substance and will suffer severe mental and physical symptoms if it is stopped. Sometimes the metabolism of the body is so altered that the addict can tolerate enormous doses of drug which would inevitably be fatal in a normal person. At this point the individual has become a true addict and his whole life is likely to be dominated by the need for the drug and the effort to obtain it.

Four general groups of drugs are particularly important in their ability to produce habituation and addiction. These groups are:

1. Hypnotic and tranquillizing drugs, including a large number of sleeping tablets, sedatives, and calming agents.
2. Euphoriant substances: the "pep-pills".
3. Hallucinogens: drugs which induce visions and produce marked alterations in sensory appreciation.
4. Analgesic substances: the powerful pain-killing drugs.

With all of these drugs habituation may occur after a prolonged period of use under medical prescription. Habituation and addiction can also occur as a result of self-administration and, as is well known, the growing problem of addiction to the opiate analgesics is currently giving rise to a good deal of alarm in this country. Amongst certain young people, drug-taking has become an acceptable custom and sometimes even a cult. They may restrict their activities to smoking hashish or to taking occasional pep-pills and most of them do not progress any further than this. People who take these "soft" drugs usually claim that they are no more tempted than the ordinary person to move on to the more dangerous drugs of addiction and it is still a matter of some controversy as to whether the pathway from "soft" to "hard" drugs is an important one. It is also argued that the social side-effects of mild drug-taking are considerably less disturbing than drunkenness and alcoholism, and yet few people are nowadays prepared to call for the prohibition of alcohol. We would argue that it is well known that habituation to drugs can be a very severe problem indeed, and since it is usually the most vulnerable and least stable young people who are tempted to use and subsequently abuse drugs, it is wrong to be permissive about their non-medical use. We appreciate that if we are not prepared to advocate the banishing of alcohol it is not strictly logical to call for a repressive attitude towards drug-taking. The problem of addiction in Britain is still relatively small but it is increasing, and the extent of the drug-habituation problem is largely unknown. The effects of severe addiction are so abominable that it is utterly wrong in our view to condone an attitude of mind which could allow addiction to become commoner. The non-medical use of drugs should be discouraged and banned, but as well as this, it is important that all those connected with the medical field should be at pains to stop fostering the impression that pills are some sort of universal panacea. It must be recognized that some degree of unhappiness is part of the human condition and can be dealt with by means other than drugs.

It is impossible to predict who may become a drug addict, just as it is impossible to say which heavy drinker will eventually become an alcoholic. However, it can certainly be said that individuals with severely disturbed personalities or psychopathy or those with long-standing neurotic symptoms are more likely than average to take drugs to excess and, once taking them, will have much more difficulty in stopping them. In general, the person who is unwilling or unable to face problems or decisions and who prefers to avoid them by seeking some form of chemical comfort is in a vulnerable position. The more disturbed the personality, the easier it is to become addicted to any substance and the individual who abuses both alcohol and drugs is often an utterly intractable therapeutic problem.

Let us now consider the different groups of addictive drugs and their various effects.

1. *Hypnotics and Tranquillizers*

Of this group, the various barbiturate drugs are the commonest substances to produce habituation and addiction. They are prescribed in considerable quantities for day-time use as sedatives and night-time use as sleeping tablets, and large amounts are consumed illegally by young people as an adjuvant to, or substitute for, alcohol. They are effective tranquillizers but have the disadvantage of causing a good deal of drowsiness. As already described, their effect may be cumulative so that the full amount of drug is not cleared from the body by the time the next dose is taken and after a period there is a considerable accumulation within the body. Eventually this may lead to marked intoxication, with unsteadiness of the gait, slurring of speech and even confusion.

The person is usually unwilling to give up the drug because he tends not to associate it with its side-effects and he prefers to avoid the risk of having the anxiety and sleeplessness return. If the extent of intoxication is not appreciated by the doctor and if the barbiturate is suddenly withdrawn, quite severe abstinence symptoms, not unlike delirium tremens, may appear. These include tremor, anxiety, headache, vertigo and vomiting. In some cases there are severe epileptic seizures a day or two after the drug is stopped, after which the patient may return to normal or may proceed to a more severe delirious state which takes some time to clear up. It is often not appreciated how dependent on a drug a patient is and he is unlikely to admit that he has increased the dose on his own initiative. If the barbiturate is suddenly stopped, perhaps because the general practitioner has become alarmed by the amount the patient is consuming, or because the patient takes ill and is admitted to hospital, or because an illegal supply has run out, the first indication of anything untoward may be the unexpected occurrence of an epileptic fit. Sometimes a relative knows that the patient is taking too many tablets and in this case the social history may alert the physician to the dangers of sudden drug-withdrawal.

An individual who is addicted to barbiturates and who cannot be weaned from them in a simple fashion must be admitted to hospital and be prevented from having access to illicit supplies. The drugs are gradually withdrawn and precautions are taken to ensure that no ill-effects occur. Then the treatment for the under-lying psychiatric condition may proceed.

There are numerous other hypnotic drugs apart from barbiturates. Most of the newer ones have been produced in an attempt to avoid the habituating effects of barbiturate and some are certainly very safe. A variety of tranquillizing drugs are also available which avoid the complication of excessive drowsiness and are relatively non-addictive. However, if a patient is sufficiently neurotic or disturbed he is capable of becoming addicted to almost anything. It is always wise to prescribe very cautiously for these people and to avoid drugs which produce any degree of euphoria or excessively pleasurable relaxation. When addiction has occurred the treatment approach is very much as for the barbiturate addict.

2. *Euphoriant Drugs*

These are a widely divergent group of substances which have the common property of producing a feeling of elation or euphoria. They also give a sensation of increased energy and temporarily reduce the need for sleep, so that they have been widely used as "pep-pills" to combat fatigue and drowsiness in members of the armed forces and in others whose occupation demands constant alertness. They are sometimes employed to treat depressive symptoms, but this effect is usually temporary and much less specific than it is in those drugs which are truly antidepressant in their action. Some of the euphoriant drugs have the side-effect of reducing appetite and they may be used to aid the process of slimming. Unfortunately all of these substances have a definite tendency to cause habituation, and since their euphoriant effect becomes less marked with continual ingestion, the dose is often raised again and again by the patient till he is taking relatively enormous quantities. Not uncommonly, euphoriants are taken in combination with barbiturates in order to achieve stimulation with calmness: the result is often addiction to both drugs.

There is no good evidence that the decrease in appetite produced by these drugs is more effective in the long run in reducing weight than simply keeping to a properly controlled diet. Nowadays, with modern antidepressant treatment there is little or no call to treat depression with euphoriants. However, amphetamine, dexamphetamine and similar drugs are still widely prescribed to stimulate jaded housewives and enable teenagers to live over-hectic lives. There is a very large black market in them and some individuals consume huge amounts of stimulants, with various ill-effects.

The rapid increase in tolerance is very striking in some people. After a time the over-stimulated individual becomes irritable and tired and of course he probably takes more tablets to counteract these feelings. Marked mood-swings may follow and there may be periods of mild confusion, especially if alcohol is taken in conjunction with the drug. There are not infrequently physical side-effects, and the blood-pressure can become raised in certain patients. Sometimes, continued taking of the euphoriant can cause a psychotic illness which closely resembles paranoid schizophrenia. This may become very severe and its symptoms include hallucinations, delusions and ideas of persecution. This condition usually resolves when the drug is withdrawn, but treatment in hospital is necessary because of the individual's disturbed behaviour and his tendency to go on secretly taking the drug and thus prolonging his symptoms. In a few cases the illness is permanent.

Cocaine is an even more seriously addictive drug which is rarely taken alone but usually in combination with one of the opiates. It may be inhaled through the nose or taken by injection. Its effect is to produce sensations of ecstatic emotion and omnipotence and the individual, though often apparently lethargic, has a feeling of superhuman energy. The effects are very short-lived and the drug is extremely addictive, so administration has to be repeated every few hours. Serious physical and mental side-effects are common and include convulsions, intolerable itching of the skin and, at times, severe delusions. The cure rate in cocainism is extremely low and the death-rate, from intoxication, infection (from unsterilized needles) and exhaustion, is high.

Hashish, or marijuana, is usually taken by inhaling the smoke of a "reefer" cigarette. It too produces euphoria and as well as this a feeling of detachment in time and space. There is a good deal of argument as to whether this drug is addictive. In most cases it appears not to be, though some disturbed individuals come to depend on it for peace of mind and as a result they lead inert and unproductive existences. Its main danger is that it frequently provides the first experience of drug-taking which in some cases leads to experimentation with more addictive drugs. Since hashish is not usually habituating there is rarely need for treatment for the taking of it. On the other hand, if the individual is using it in a compulsive way his underlying psychiatric disorder may need attention, and since this type of person is quite frequently a social misfit his problem may require considerable help from the social worker.

3. *The Hallucinogens*

These drugs have various effects, but one of the most prominent is that they produce visual hallucinations. They also produce distortions of sensation, including disturbance of orientation in time and space and alteration of appreciation of the self and of one's body image. Sometimes they induce ecstatic mood-states and this effect is sought in the religious ceremonies of some primitive peoples who have discovered the hallucinogenic effects of certain plants. The hallucinogens include Lysergic Acid Diethylamide (L.S.D. 25), Mescaline, Psilocybin and others. In recent years they have been used by some psychiatrists to facilitate the release of unconscious material during psychotherapy, but this has not come to be widely practised and there is no convincing proof that this method of treatment has any specifically valuable effects. The hallucinogens are also used by certain semi-mystical cults in our society in order to undergo "transcendental" experiences which are really confusional states with accompanying distortions of sensory impressions. These may be pleasant but in some people are very frightening and may precipitate quite severe psychiatric disorders. The hallucinogenic drugs can become addictive, and in addition to this they may cause the individual to behave in very strange ways while he is under their influence: for instance, it has been reported that several people have become convinced after taking L.S.D. that they could fly and have jumped to their deaths while suffering from this delusion.

In view of the lack of clear-cut usefulness in the therapeutic field and the possibly dangerous side-effects, we believe that this group of drugs should be available only for properly conducted psychological experiments.

4. *The Opiates*

In Britain, the problem of addiction to these drugs is still relatively small, but even so, there has been an alarming upsurge in the past few years. Previously, the greater proportion of addicts in this country consisted of people from the medical or para-medical professions who had ready access to drugs, or individuals who had become addicted as a result of opiate treatment for prolonged and severely painful conditions. Nowadays most of the new cases of addiction arise as a result of illegal drug-trafficking and they occur mostly in young people.

Drugs such as morphine and heroin are profoundly addictive. They produce a relaxed, drowsy state with mild euphoria and with pleasant fantasies and dreams. Some individuals seem to be able to take the drug intermittently without having any particular withdrawal effects when they stop, but most addicts, especially those taking heroin, soon find that they need more and more of the drug to maintain even a semblance of well-being. Life becomes a compulsive search for it with every other activity subordinated to the need to find money for the next dose. Often the person cannot afford to work and if he is getting the heroin illegally he may have to steal to get sufficient funds. Most of his money goes on the drug and so malnutrition is common. As heroin is usually taken by injection and sterile precautions are rarely observed, the addict often has severe skin infections and he sometimes develops jaundice because dirty needles can transmit the virus of infective hepatitis. The combined effects of the drug, his poor general condition, undernourishment and irregular living conditions frequently lead to severe physical illness and the death-rate among opiate addicts is very high indeed.

In opiate addiction terrifying symptoms usually follow withdrawal of the drug and the addict has no desire to experience these, so he goes on taking ever-bigger doses. If the drug is stopped and no treatment is given the patient develops mild restlessness, yawning and vague feelings of discomfort after about 12 hours. After this he experiences severe aches all over his body, general feelings of malaise, fever and complete insomnia. These symptoms progress to extreme restlessness, severe nausea and feelings of intense fear and horror. The peak is usually reached after about 48 hours and the symptoms then gradually pass off, though vague feelings of unwellness may persist for a considerable time. All of these symptoms are rapidly relieved by an adequate dose of the appropriate drug and there is little wonder that a further injection of the opiate is much preferred by the addict even if it means continued enslavement to drug-taking.

Heroin addicts are often addicted to cocaine and, in some of the worst cases, to alcohol as well. Many addicts have very inadequate psychological resources at the best of times and this tends to produce very poor results when treatment is attempted. Their way of life is irregular and their personal attitudes may be abhorrent to many people. It is admittedly difficult to be sympathetic with many heroin addicts and it is sometimes suggested that since they have elected to be like this they should be allowed to live (and die) as they choose. We do not share this view. We deprecate the frame of mind that leads an individual to become dependent on drugs, but we must recognize that the addict is a very sick person who requires treatment if he is to have a reasonable chance of continuing to remain alive. We urgently need to acquire more effective means of treating individual cases of addiction, but, in addition, society must learn to tackle the problem in general very quickly lest the whole situation get out of hand as has happened, for example, in the United States.

Until the recent passing of the Dangerous Drugs (Supply to Addicts) Act (1968), all medical practitioners in Britain were entitled to prescribe opiate drugs to known addicts at their own discretion and this system worked well for many years. With the rapid increase in the number of addicts the situation began to get out of control, and under the new regulations addicts may be supplied with opiates only by specially licensed practitioners who have experience in dealing with such patients. Treatment is to be carried out to a great extent in special Addiction Units, details of the treatment varying somewhat from place to place according to the experience of the doctor in charge. The aim is always to get the patient completely off the drug, but if this is not possible an attempt is made to reduce the dosage to more reasonable levels. Sometimes the drug is withdrawn gradually, by slowly tapering the doses, but in the view of some specialists it is better to stop the heroin suddenly and prevent the severe withdrawal effects by means of very heavy sedation. Along with this treatment it is nearly always necessary to improve the patient's extremely debilitated physical state.

Co-operation from the addict is often half-hearted at best and the relapse rate is invariably high. The individual has usually become an outcast from his family, and if treatment is to be successful the members of the household must be persuaded to re-accept him. The outlook is better where the family is a stable one, but too often there is a background of a broken or inadequate home. The addict who has responded well to treatment needs a great deal of help in finding and keeping work, making new social contacts and forming stable interpersonal relationships. This is often a prolonged process, even in successful cases, because the patient frequently lacks initiative and adequate motivation. Often the struggle proves too much for the addict and relapse occurs, but intensive treatment and social work which concentrates on rendering the environment less stressful do lessen the chances of relapse.

Note

The prevention of drug addiction is a vital problem for our society. It seems incredible to the average person that anyone could start on the path that leads to drug-dependence when it is well known what the end result is likely to be. Unhappily, it is usually the weak, the disturbed and those who lack foresight who are likely to mis-use drugs and who become irretrievably "hooked". As much as the treatment of the addicted individual, it is necessary to deal with the illicit organizations which promote addiction and tempt the cured addict to relapse. This may necessitate close co-operation between the staff of an addiction unit, social workers and outside agencies, including the police. The drug addict who is receiving treatment is very much our patient or client and his rights must be respected, but it is to his advantage as much as to anyone else's that the traffic in drugs be brought to an end. Addiction is too dreadful a price to pay for being excessively permissive in our social attitudes and indiscriminate drug-taking must be whole-heartedly condemned and prevented.

CHAPTER 8

Suicide and Attempted Suicide

WHEN we have been discussing the various psychiatric illnesses we have indicated that some of them carry a greater risk of suicidal behaviour than others. But it is important at the outset of this topic to emphasize that such behaviour is a complex phenomenon and does not occur only in relation to mental illnesses. We believe that it is a separate entity which sometimes occurs in the setting of a psychiatric disorder, but in order to understand it fully a variety of personal, social and demographic factors must be taken into account.

Suicide is one of the four legal categories of mode of death (the others being death due to homicide, accident and natural causes) and the layman usually assumes that, in order to commit suicide, some positive action must be taken by the individual, such as taking an overdose of drugs, shooting or drowning himself. Data on comparative rates for suicide as a means of death are based on this assumption despite the fact that a dictionary would probably be less specific and would describe a suicide as "one who kills himself intentionally". According to this definition suicide can be an act of omission as well as of commission, and the patient who fails to take a life-saving drug (for example, the diabetic who neglects to give himself his vital injections of insulin) may be intentionally trying to end his life. However, if he were successful in killing himself it is unlikely that his death would be included in the suicide statistics as it does not come within the traditional definition of the act. A further confusion often arises even when a person does take active steps to harm himself and dies as a result of his action, because the coroner or other official may decide that there was no real "intent" to die and a verdict such as "death by misadventure" may be recorded.

The concept of attempted suicide also is frequently confused by the vagaries of semantics and of official attitudes but, from our point of view, it is important (as with suicide) to determine "intent" in order to understand the patient and the course of action he has pursued. "Attempted suicide" is neither a definition nor a diagnosis, but instead represents an interpretation of an act. If we decide too hastily and without investigation that a person who has taken an overdose of drugs, or committed some other potentially self-destructive deed, was attempting to end his life, then we are likely to be blind to the possibility that perhaps he was not seeking death. The subsequent handling of a case which has been wrongly interpreted in this way would most likely be inappropriate and possibly even harmful to the individual.

Many writers and research workers have attempted to define suicidal behaviour in such a way as to remove some of the confusion which surrounds it, but no one, so far as we know, has succeeded in providing a definition which satisfies all the psychological, sociological and legal criteria which are involved. We find it necessary to stress that these difficulties of definition exist in order that the reader will be fully aware that present-day statistics of suicide and attempted suicide are very far from being accurate. It is also unfortunately true that the results of different research studies on the subject cannot be satisfactorily compared with each other in many instances since comparable definitions and methods have not been used by the investigators. The widely varying results that have been found in different places and at different times have given rise to much theoretical speculation which is often quite groundless because they are based largely on statistical artefact.

In view of all these difficulties of assessment it is clear that whatever figures are calculated for suicide are likely to be underestimates. Suicidal behaviour is obviously a matter for serious concern, the more so when we realize that, no matter how large the problem appears in the published statistics, the real facts would be likely to be even more drastic if they could be accurately estimated. In Great

Britain about 5500 people are recorded as having committed suicide each year—that is, about one person per ten thousand of the population per annum. However, as we have indicated, the actual figure is possibly much higher. Cross-cultural comparisons are interesting but are difficult to make for the reasons we have mentioned and also because the methods of recording vital statistics vary widely according to the stage of social development attained by a community. It is certain, however, that each year the equivalent of a city the size of Geneva kills itself. Despite our present ignorance we can say that there probably are culturally determined differences in suicide rates. Primitive races are thought to have lower rates than those found in more highly developed societies and, according to Durkheim's (1897) theory, the rates should vary inversely with the degree of cohesion within a society. Certainly in time of war when, amongst other things, national cohesiveness is at its highest, the incidence of suicide tends to diminish. There is also some evidence that where there are minority groups living in the midst of another culture their rates for suicide are frequently lower than the rates for the predominant population. As regards "attempted suicide", it will be apparent from what we have already said that its incidence depends on many variables, not the least of these being the way in which we define the phenomenon. In general it is accepted that the rates for attempted suicide in modern Western communities may be as much as twenty times greater than those for completed suicide.

We do not propose to develop the theme of cultural comparisons, nor do we wish to inflict on our readers a mass of statistical data. We are particularly concerned to show the seriousness of this problem and to discuss it in such a way that the social worker may comprehend some of its complexities and also be able to deal more competently with the suicidal patient when she comes in contact with him in the course of her work. We have stressed the difficulties of definition, but clearly the field worker must have some basic guide-lines to help her, and to make matters as simple as possible we shall present a description of suicide and attempted suicide based on the premise that a person who acts in this way has an underlying wish to destroy, harm or injure himself. We see suicidal behaviour as a continuum with the desire for death at one end and, at the other, an attempt to call attention to unhappiness but with no real wish to die. Between these extremes can be observed many serious activities which include varying degrees and combinations of non-lethal self-injury (or threats of it) with varying degrees of seriousness of intent.

Suicidal activity is usually impulsive, the thought being rapidly translated into action. But the thought necessarily includes the element of intent, and if we are to understand where the individual patient fits on our continuum we must endeavour to assess the nature of this intent as accurately as we can. Clearly there may be a substantial difference in the expected outcome in the person who takes a large overdose of drugs in the presence of others as compared with that in the individual who takes a similar overdose in the seclusion of his own room. The seriousness of the attempt cannot simply be assessed by what the patient took or did. We must also take into consideration the precautions he observed to ensure or to avoid discovery and the psychological state in which he was at the time the attempt was made. For example, we mention elsewhere (see p. 206) that people who are severely depressed are a high risk group for suicide. These patients may have a very definite wish for death and yet, because their illness causes retardation of thought and deed, the action which they take to achieve self-destruction may be poorly planned. Sometimes they lack initiative to do any-thing, but if they do attempt suicide it is often insufficient to cause death. Even if the attempt was potentially lethal the patient's social constellation may be so closely knit that discovery before death would be almost certain. In the circumstances one could well gain the impression that the suicidal behaviour was more of a gesture than a real attempt and this might be a very grave error of judgement.

One of the great dangers in this field is that when the individual's action appears to be insufficient to achieve his total destruction we automatically consign him to one of two categories. We assume either that he was not really trying to harm himself or else that he was trying to die and, having failed in his attempt, will certainly try again. Most suicidal people do not fall into such neat categories because very often they themselves are not completely clear about their own motives. They "gamble" with death in such a way that consciously or unconsciously they place on others the responsibility for the decision as to whether they live or die. Many people who have a sincere wish to die and who attempt to destroy themselves are only suicidal for a limited time and if their act is unsuccessful they may never repeat their suicidal behaviour, but not all individuals who survive fall into this group. There is good evidence that some people are "repeat prone" and it has been shown that this is particularly true of individuals with personality disorders, particularly if this is coupled with addiction to alcohol or drugs or both. It is also true of some of the people we have already described who failed on the first occasion because of temporary lack of volition. When treatment has produced slight improvement, depression may still be present, but initiative is sufficiently recovered to allow the patient to put his morbid thoughts into action. Especial vigilance is therefore necessary during the early stages of recovery.

A common fallacy is the belief that people who talk about suicide rarely commit it, but there is danger in ignoring suicide threats. It has been found that at least eight out of every ten people who kill themselves give quite definite warning of their intent. Although the act itself may be impulsive, the suicidal individual usually tells other people that he will kill himself and these remarks must be heeded. We do not say that we should allow ourselves to be manipulated by the threat, but we must not ignore it.

There are various other fallacies about suicidal behaviour which are current. For example, it is often said that it is peculiarly likely to occur in the upper social classes, but as Shneidman and Farberow (1957) have said, "Suicide is neither the rich man's disease nor the poor man's curse. Suicide is very 'democratic' and is represented proportionately among all levels of society." It is sometimes believed that "suicide is inherited" or that it "runs in a family". We do not believe that suicide can be inherited because it seems to be a form of behaviour whose causation is multifactorial. However, we certainly cannot ignore the influence of the family, and genetic factors may certainly be involved when, for example, depressive illness occurs in successive generations. Along with depression often goes the risk of suicide and it may be this which causes the seeming "inheritance" of suicide. Also, it is known that persons with personality abnormalities are excessively liable to display suicidal behaviour, and since their children not infrequently develop similar character-traits it is not surprising that they too should form a high risk group. In this latter type of case, the abnormalities of personality and the tendency to suicide may be both related to the lack of stable and consistent emotional relationships during the individual's early upbringing. Another false belief is the one which declares that everyone who behaves in a suicidal fashion is mentally ill. In fact, many people who attempt to kill themselves are unhappy rather than unwell. Severe distress is not synonymous with psychiatric disorder even when it reaches such a pitch that it is completely overwhelming. If at this instant the means of suicide is at hand the person may impulsively reach for it in a desperate attempt to escape from unbearable tension.

Shneidman and Farberow are outstanding authorities in this field and they have described four main types of suicidal crisis as follows:

1. *Impulsive suicidal behaviour* in the heat of anger, disappointment or frustration, which is usually of a temporary nature but should nevertheless be recognized as a dangerous manifestation which could lead to tragedy.

2. *The feeling that life is no longer worth living* may appear when a person has come to believe, over a period of time, that life is meaningless or that he is no longer wanted or needed. Sometimes he feels that his difficulties are insurmountable and that it is pointless to go on.

3. *Very serious illness*, when the individual who is in constant pain or who believes that he has an incurable disease sees death as an escape from suffering.

4. *"Communication" suicide attempts*, where the underlying motive is to convey a message or to attempt to change the behaviour of other people rather than to die. This form of behaviour constitutes a gamble, and if the plan for rescue goes wrong the individual may become an accidental suicide.

How may the suicide-prone person be identified before he reaches the stage of committing the act? It is very likely that he will communicate his intentions either by saying directly that he will kill himself or else by some form of unusual behaviour such as getting his affairs in order, sometimes in a rather conspicuous and meaningful way. A seeming lack of concern about whether he lives or dies is often significant, as are feelings of hopelessness which are frequently expressed quite freely. Many of the clues which are most useful to us relate to the illness entities which carry a high risk of suicide. For example, symptoms of a depressive illness such as feelings of dejection and guilt, physical or psychological exhaustion, hopelessness, loss of interest in work, hobbies or sex and so on are always worthy of serious attention. When the depression occurs in a setting of alcoholism, personality disorder, psychopathy or a combination of these conditions the risk of suicide is very high indeed.

The impending suicidal crisis requires a rapid appraisal in order to assess just how dangerous is the possibility of acting-out behaviour, and with this need in view we cautiously offer a number of additional criteria which may help in evaluating imminent suicidal potential. It has been suggested in the past that elderly males carry the highest risk, but recent investigations have indicated that though cultural variables occur, there appears to be an approximately equal risk for the two sexes. However, two high risk age groups seem to emerge from the statistics. The first consists of elderly people who have suffered bereavement or who live alone, who are lonely, have perhaps fallen on hard times and who receive little or no social support. The second is a younger group, consisting of individuals suffering from personality disorders coupled with addiction to alcohol or drugs, and these we have already mentioned above. In both these groups there are some important indications of immediate risk. For example, the more specific the suicidal plans the greater is the danger. A history of previous suicidal behaviour tends to add to the current risk, but it is doubtful if the seriousness of earlier attempts gives much help, partly because of the difficulty of assessing seriousness, partly because the individual is often pharmacologically unsophisticated and has no idea of what constitutes an overdose, and partly because of (as we have previously described) a lack of volition due to illness. If physical complaints are present they may sometimes be masking an underlying depressive illness. Recent bereavement or loss by separation or divorce or the anniversary of such a loss not uncommonly appears to precipitate depression and a desire to rejoin the loved one. If the potential suicide remains in contact with a sympathetic environment the risk is diminished, but the risk is greatly increased if the environment is a rejecting one. We may infer from this that the patient is likely to benefit from a social worker who is prepared to listen, be sympathetic and helpful and knows when to seek appropriate help from the psychiatrist or physician. Simply allowing the patient to communicate his distress may avert a crisis. However, a word of warning is necessary. Some suicides very successfully conceal their intent and this is sometimes a feature of the illness which underlies the desire for death in these particular patients. The social worker who has been conscientious in her approach to the patient and who has sought the psychiatrist's advice when necessary must not blame herself unduly when, as inevitably occurs, the occasional suicide occurs despite all her efforts.

Theories of the Causation of Suicidal Behaviour

These theories tend to be either sociological or psychological and semantic disagreements between the two camps lead to much fruitless argument. Emile Durkheim (1897), whose work is still widely quoted, favoured the sociological view, believing that suicide was largely dependent on the pressures exerted by certain social forces and that the greater the degree of social cohesion, the lower would be the risk of suicide. Some recent studies have lent some support to his assertions by showing that where there are problems due to breakdown of close interpersonal relationships as, for example, the broken home, marital disharmony or love problems, the risk of suicidal behaviour is high. Other social problems of a wider nature have also been demonstrated to have an association with suicide and these may also be indices of low social cohesiveness.

They include financial problems, which sometimes constitute a specific precipitating factor and sometimes indicate a chronic state of impoverishment, with consequent loss of morale; employment problems, including fears of dismissal or redundancy; crime and the fear of pursuit and prosecution. These evidences of the individual's social difficulties may of course result from aberrations of personality and need not of themselves be causally related to suicide. Without belittling the significance of long-term adverse social factors in the precipitation of suicidal behaviour we must point out that these are usually not sufficient to account entirely for such a severe reaction.

The presence of adverse social factors often tells us as much about the suicidal person's personality as about the motivation for the act itself. Whatever the individual's social circumstances, the act is that of a unique human being and to understand it fully we must also invoke psychological explanations. Broadly speaking, these are derived from either psychoanalytic or non-psychoanalytic schools of thought. The psychoanalytic viewpoint is largely based on Freud's concept of the psychodynamics of depression and his postulation of the existence of a death instinct. It therefore tends to equate suicidal behaviour with mental illness. Recent research of a non-doctrinaire type has shown that this is not necessarily so and has demonstrated that it is only too easy to assume that depression must be present because suicide has been attempted. If one is determined to believe in the overwhelming importance of psychiatric illness one can argue that attempted suicide has an emotionally cathartic effect so that symptoms present at the time of the actual act may have subsided before the doctor can interview the patient. However, careful psychiatric and social histories taken soon after the attempt often fail to reveal evidence of psychiatric abnormality and it is not permissible simply to infer that a hypothetical illness has come and gone.

No one theory can account for the complexities of suicidal behaviour. In any case, there has been a good deal too much theorizing and not enough scientific work on the subject. Fortunately this is now beginning to alter for the better.

The Social History in Attempted Suicide

When a suicide attempt has occurred and the patient has survived, the initial medical treatment is nowadays usually carried out in hospital. Once the immediate danger is past it is necessary to plan the therapeutic approach and a good social history is of great value for diagnosis, prognosis and for the formulation of the treatment plan. In Chapter 4 we described a schema for a standard social history, but in the case of attempted suicide there is a good deal of additional information which must be obtained before the significance of the act can be adequately assessed. For example, in the case of a drug overdose it is important to ascertain which drug was used, where it was obtained, how much of it was taken and how much was left.

In attempted suicide in general, the following points should be noted:

1. Was the patient unconscious at any time following the attempt?
2. Did the patient give any indications of intent and, if so, were these recognized and acted upon by others?
3. Was there any degree of premeditation in the act itself?
4. Can a motive be discerned and was there any precipitating event?
5. Had there been any previous suicidal attempts?
6. How was the patient discovered and by whom, and who effected his admission to hospital?
7. What were the circumstances in which the attempt occurred and what steps did the patient take to ensure or avoid discovery?
8. Had the patient been drinking alcohol prior to the attempt?
9. In what way have the key relatives or acquaintances reacted to the occurrence?
10. Any other information which may be relevant.

The Treatment Approach in Attempted Suicide

It is advisable to take the history as soon after the event as possible. This is partly because the information will be fresher and partly because treatment can be more quickly initiated. Attempted suicide is often a form of communication and involves the individual's special acquaintances. Your key informant is nearly always closely embroiled in the situation and at the time of the attempt he stands in an especially meaningful relationship to the patient. The therapeutic team must quickly recognize the special needs of these two people so that the situation can be exploited to their greatest advantage at a time when they are most likely to accept advice. Preferably, the evaluation of the patient and the initiation of therapy or practical help should be carried out while the patient is in hospital since there is always a possibility that, once she leaves hospital, she will encounter the same stressful situations but may no longer be prepared to do something constructive about them. The act of attempting suicide usually causes a temporary disruption of the habitual relationship between the patient and the key acquaintance and both are likely to experience anxiety, guilt and remorse. At this point there is an unrivalled opportunity to step in with treatment before the old emotional situation reasserts itself and also to try to alter any adverse material circumstances which have been causing distress. It is usually useless to try to treat the patient as an entity in herself and in order to help her to the greatest extent we must bring the other partner into the therapeutic situation. The value of involving the key person immediately is given some support by recent research findings which showed that after the event the social situation improved most often when close interpersonal relations improved. Conversely, the patients whose social situation deteriorated were more often found to be those whose close relationships had either remained unsatisfactory or had deteriorated even further.

Although we have suggested that a suicidal attempt may be an act which is aimed at altering the behaviour of the key person, improvement in the relationship after the act is more likely to be related to alteration in the behaviour of the attempter also. Patients who have the poorest prognosis are generally those who have the greatest difficulty in their interpersonal relationships, and this is especially so in the case of a married person when either she or her husband have expressed a desire to end the marriage before the suicide attempt was made.

Another important reason which makes it desirable to contact relatives as soon after the event as possible is that frequently the key person may be more in need of help than the patient. Earlier we pointed out that a suicidal attempt could occur because of extreme unhappiness rather than as a result of mental illness, and we have indicated just how intense this unhappiness can be when, for example, the attempter is married to an individual with an affectionless personality. It is important in the treatment plan to know how much support can be obtained from the environment and to be able to assess this quickly so that treatment is not delayed.

We have indicated that suicidal behaviour may occur entirely as a result of mental illness and when the illness is alleviated there is little more for the psychiatrist and social worker to do. However, when the patient suffers from a character disorder, especially if coupled with an addiction to drugs or alcohol, and the act appears to have been precipitated by social events, the treatment plan becomes much more complex. We have pointed out that it may be very unrewarding for the social worker to work with these difficult personalities and yet, in terms of suicide, they constitute a very high risk group of people. In Chapter 6 we described the aetiology of psychopathy and indicated that one of the most important causal factors in this disorder was a disturbed early upbringing. We believe that although "cure" may be difficult, if not impossible, prevention of the development of such personalities may not be, and recent research into the reasons for suicide and attempted suicide has indicated that it may be possible to identify this very high risk group of individuals from a very early age and therefore at a time when intervention may be more rewarding. Persons who behave in a suicidal way have an abnormally high rate of contact in their childhood with agencies who deal with cruelty to children;

with departments who have responsibility for child welfare; and with school authorities who are concerned with truancy. It seems likely that appropriate, though perhaps prolonged, social support and treatment applied in these early stages may be much more rewarding in the long run.

It is worth stressing that there are many character-disordered adults who attempt suicide who are yet capable of maturing into responsible citizens. Though we have indicated that for many the prognosis is poor, we believe that if even a few of them can be helped it is worth while to make the effort to rehabilitate them. However, so long as social workers have, because of the size of their case-load, to allocate their time carefully they must consider how much effort they can invest in these cases in relation to the cost to other patients. It is not realistic to think of solving the problems which surround patients with abnormal personalities in a few weeks or months. However, anyone who has deliberately poisoned or injured himself but survived must be made aware that there is always help available without his having to resort to this dangerous form of behaviour to receive it. This must be a sincere offer backed, if at all possible, by the availability of a hospital bed for those who need sanctuary while the risk of a suicide attempt is high.

We have discussed some of the main prognostic indicators and we would emphasize that the social ones are at least as important as the clinical ones. What is *not* important is the act itself or even the immediate precipitating factors. The act is far less of a guide to the subsequent social outcome than the normal background setting of the individual. The apparent seriousness is not a good guide since experience has taught us that many people who, at a first attempt, do not seriously endanger their lives do in fact subsequently kill themselves. Conversely, many people whose attempts very seriously endangered their lives never again behave suicidally. Attempted suicide is the result of a process; that process may be an illness, some abnormality of personality development, or a series of social factors and it is wrong that management of the patient should be determined only by the "seriousness" of the attempt. Treatment of the patient should be decided by the clinical state of the patient and his usual, rather than his immediate, social situation.

By far the most important factor which is associated with social and/or marital improvement is the alteration of the attitude and behaviour of the patient and any key person associated with the act towards each other. This is especially true of the person who has attempted suicide, for when her behaviour towards the key person remains static or worsens, subsequent improvement in her more general social setting is very rare indeed.

CHAPTER 9

The Functional Psychoses

THESE are the severe mental disorders in which no evidence of underlying organic brain dysfunction has been proved to exist. (Many psychiatrists would say "has not yet been proved" as there is a strong feeling that there may be underlying biochemical abnormalities.) The two main categories of illness here are the Affective Disorders and Schizophrenia: apart from being grouped together to make a neat classification, these illnesses appear to be quite independent of each other.

A. THE AFFECTIVE DISORDERS

The word "Affect" is used more or less synonymously with the word "Emotion", and the affective illnesses show an abnormality of mood as their predominant pathological feature. The abnormality may consist of excessive sadness or excessive cheerfulness and in some cases an element of pathological anxiety may be present.

Mood

Before considering these illnesses in detail it is worth while mentioning the way in which mood may normally vary. We all have a mood-state which (if we think of it at all) we regard as normal and we know that this can be influenced in various ways. Good news may make us feel happy, even overjoyed, whereas a sad event tends to make us dejected or depressed. Sometimes the event which has caused the mood-change occurs within us rather than outside: for example, we may wake up unduly cheerful after a pleasant dream or the thought of some impending event which we fear (for example, the examination for which we have not adequately prepared) may make us very unhappy. No matter how our mood-state is affected, we know that in normal circumstances it will always show a tendency to return to a normal base-line.

Different people seem to have base-lines which are set at different levels. We know that some individuals are habitually more cheerful and others are consistently more pessimistic than we ourselves are. All of us are continually reacting to our environment in our own particular ways, experiencing events which make us momentarily happier or sadder, and we tend to think of our mood-level as a kind of barometer which registers the way circumstances are treating us at any particular time.

However, there are times when we are unaccountably sad or happy, very much as though our mood was temporarily reacting independently of external events. Sometimes the mood-swing is caused by a thought or a recollection, but on occasion we may be particularly aware that our affective state is not appropriate to events outside or inside ourselves. This may happen when we have one of these unaccountable "moods" which are not at all uncommon. This type of feeling usually passes quite quickly and we usually put it down to an attack of indigestion or liverishness or something like that. But there are some people who are more likely than the rest of us to experience such moods: their emotional state shows a tendency to be labile and they may become more easily elated or more easily dejected than the average person. Sometimes when this happens, they take longer than normal to return to a normal state of equilibrium. This phenomenon is common enough to be regarded usually as a normal variant and we talk about such people as exhibiting a "cyclothymic" type of personality, that is, they are particularly subject to mood-swings.

Most cyclothymic individuals are perfectly normal people, but a proportion of them do show a tendency to pathological mood-swings and occasionally in one of these they will slip into an affective type of illness which then appears to be simply an exaggeration or prolongation of their usual mood-change. There are variations on the cyclothymic personality: for example, there are people who are almost permanently over-active and cheerful and others who are always rather pessimistic in their attitudes. Where these characteristics are very prominent it is thought that the individuals concerned probably have a somewhat increased risk of developing an affective disorder.

Classification of Affective Illness

The commonest form of affective disorder is Depressive Illness. This may occur in all degrees of severity from something that is little more than a rather severe mood-swing to an illness in which the patient suffers all the mental agonies of the damned. For simplicity's sake we shall concentrate on the severer forms of depression in this chapter and the relatively mild forms are included in the chapter dealing with the psychoneuroses (see p. 85). The feeling that we call depression is well known to all of us but, as will be shown, severe depressive illness cannot simply be understood in terms of dejection alone. Patients who have had a depressive illness will usually report when they have recovered that the illness goes beyond the quality of simple depression.

The other main form of affective illness is Mania. In this condition the patient is pathologically elated and over-excited. When it occurs in relatively mild form it is known as Hypomania.

It is impossible to know where the normal limits of mood-change stop and affective illness starts, and each individual will have his own range of normality. As will be seen, there are sometimes peculiar difficulties in diagnosing mania, but in practice it is usually not too difficult to recognize that someone is suffering from an excessive degree of depression. The following simple schema shows the relation of the affective disorders to the normal mood level.

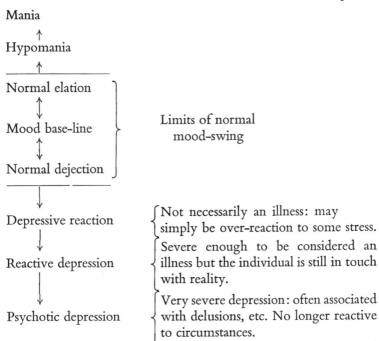

Mania
↑
Hypomania
↑

Normal elation ⎤
↑↓
Mood base-line ⎬ Limits of normal mood-swing
↑↓
Normal dejection ⎦

↓

Depressive reaction — {Not necessarily an illness: may simply be over-reaction to some stress.

↓

Reactive depression — {Severe enough to be considered an illness but the individual is still in touch with reality.

↓

Psychotic depression — {Very severe depression: often associated with delusions, etc. No longer reactive to circumstances.

The classification of depressive illness is a controversial subject and tends to confuse psychiatrists and social workers alike. The following terms are mentioned for your information, but it should not necessarily be assumed that they refer to strictly separate conditions:

(a) *Neurotic (reactive) depression.* Depression which is usually not of severe intensity and often appears to be related to environmental stresses. According to some psychiatrists it occurs more readily in unstable personalities and is often admixed with other neurotic symptoms.

(b) *Psychotic (endogenous) depression.* This illness is much more intense and is less obviously related to precipitating factors. It may be associated with severe guilt feelings, suicidal thoughts, retardation, severe anxiety and delusions of guilt and of somatic disorder.

(c) *Manic-depressive illness.* In this condition depressive illness of the endogenous type may alternate with attacks of mania or hypomania. The pattern of occurrence varies greatly and the commonest consists of recurring episodes of endogenous depression.

(d) *Involutional depression* (involutional melancholia). This term is rapidly going out of favour but is still mentioned by many text-books. It used to be thought that depressive illness occurring for the first time in middle age had a tendency to appear in people with a particular type of rather rigid personality. There is no evidence that involutional depression differs from endogenous depression.

There appears to be little or no controversy about the classification of mania.

Depressive Illness

This is a relatively common condition. Somewhere between 1 and 2 per cent of the general population will require treatment for a severe degree of depressive illness at some time in their lives and a considerably higher proportion will suffer from milder forms of depressive illness. About three women will be affected for every two men who develop the illness. It is a condition which occurs predominantly in middle and old age and it is said to be uncommon before the age of twenty, though some child psychiatrists believe that it is a relatively frequent complaint in childhood and adolescence, though it may present in disguised forms. One of the characteristics of depressive illness (particularly endogenous depression) is its tendency to recur: this tendency is not invariable and up to one-half of those who have a depressive illness never have a further attack. Fortunately the illness does not usually produce any permanent deteriorative effect on the patient's mental functioning, either intellectual or otherwise, and even if it recurs frequently, return to normality between attacks is the rule. Recurrent forms of the illness may manifest as repeated attacks of depression but sometimes the pattern is of alternating periods of depression and mania.

Depressive illness can occur in all degrees of severity and the relatively mild cases are easy to miss or mis-diagnose. The onset of the condition is often insidious and to begin with the patient is simply aware of being out-of-sorts. In these circumstances he begins to look for causes of his malaise and may start complaining in hypochondriacal fashion of various bodily symptoms which he becomes convinced are being caused by serious physical illness. If he complains persistently enough he may be sent for a specialist opinion, not to a psychiatrist but to a physician or a surgeon, because his somatic complaints have completely overshadowed the depression. Thus, cases of depression are not infrequently found at surgical and gynaecological clinics (sometimes only after they have undergone an unnecessary operation).

The majority of cases of depressive illness are not too severe and show a tendency to recover fairly quickly, perhaps within a few weeks. These patients rarely need to attend hospital. The more profound depressive illnesses cause the patient the most intense misery and are often associated with a real risk of suicide, and these people are usually admitted to hospital for observation and treatment. One's view of depressive illness depends largely on one's standpoint: the hospital-based psychiatrist tends to think of depression as a severe condition with a mortality rate due to suicide, whereas the general practitioner is more likely to see it as a relatively mild illness on the whole but with a small proportion of more severe cases whom he will usually refer to the psychiatrist.

Symptoms of Depressive Illness

In the majority of cases the most noticeable symptom will of course be depression, though sometimes, rather paradoxically, depression is not an immediately observable feature of depressive illness: for example, some cases of facial pain turn out to be due to affective illness. Where depression is obvious it may consist of mild dejection or, at the other extreme, of the most utter and inconsolable misery.

We have divided the symptoms of depressive illness into three main categories: those which are predominantly psychological, those which involve somatic complaints, and those which produce changes in the individual's social functioning.

1. *Psychological symptoms.* In milder cases of depression the mood tends to vary in intensity from time to time and often lifts temporarily in cheerful company, etc. In the more severe illnesses it shows a tendency to increase steadily in depth and to cease to react in accordance with stimuli from the environment. The patient appears sunk in despair and it is quite useless to try to talk him out of this state: he may respond slightly but soon relapses into misery again. In severer cases, retardation may be noticeable: the person's mental and physical activities are slowed up until, in extreme cases, he just sits round in a state of gloomy apathy. Feelings of self-reproach and guilt are often expressed: the patient may say he has committed some terrible sin or he may confess to misdemeanours which he did not commit. Sometimes he feels his corruption is contaminating other people around him. The world seems a wicked place: sometimes we read of a mother murdering her children and then killing herself, and often this occurs in the setting of a depressive illness. The woman, in her delusions, thinks that the world is too corrupt and she kills the children so that they do not have to suffer the pain of living in it.

Thoughts of suicide are often present in depressive illness and the severity of the illness is not necessarily a guide to the degree of suicide risk. Many depressives contemplate suicide and never attempt it, but one should never take chances. If a depressive has suicidal thoughts he is better kept under observation for his own sake. It is said that a very retarded depressive is too apathetic to kill himself, but this rule cannot always be relied upon.

In all cases of depression there is loss of the normal feeling of well-being. The patient becomes irritable and restless and he often finds it difficult to concentrate on tasks, so the man's work and the woman's housework suffer. Self-reproach inevitably follows and this is not helped by the frequent admonitions of other people to "Pull yourself together", or to "Do something about yourself". Difficulty in remembering is complained of, but this is due to lack of concentration rather than any actual defect in memory. Sometimes anxiety and agitation are a prominent part of the picture and may on occasion be so obvious that they completely overshadow the depression.

In the severest cases of depression the individual may develop delusional ideas and ideas of persecution. These usually show a marked degree of guilt in their content: for example, the patient may say that the police are following him everywhere, but that he deserves this because he has committed so many atrocious crimes.

2. *Somatic symptoms.* These often form a very prominent part of the depressive's complaints and in many instances depression first comes to the attention of a doctor when the patient arrives complaining of bodily ailments which have no determinable physical cause.

Loss of appetite is common, sometimes leading to a complete disinterest in food. Naturally, loss of weight will follow and also, because of the lack of food-intake, constipation is frequent. Patients often complain at great length about their lack of bowel-movements and they may become convinced that there is a blockage inside, probably caused by cancer. Whatever the symptoms, they will tend to put the worst construction on it. Women often complain of excessive menstrual bleeding and develop the conviction that they have cancer of the uterus.

Loss of energy is almost invariable and various aches and pains, especially headache, are common. This last will probably be interpreted as due to a brain tumour. Interest in sex wanes very considerably and in men there may be actual impotence: this often encourages the patient to think that he has contracted venereal disease, a very frequently expressed fear in depression. When the illness is severe, these somatic complaints cease to be just hypochondriacal and become delusional in their intensity. Then the patient will say that his insides are being gnawed away by maggots or his brain has rotted and turned to fluid, and at the time he fully believes in such ideas.

3. *Changes in social functioning.* As the depressive condition develops, the increasing inability to concentrate and the reduction in drive will make the patient less efficient at work. This often generates anxiety which in turn makes him even less efficient and more depressed. Judgement may be affected by the illness and this sometimes leads to rash decisions: for example, a man may suddenly

leave a job he has held down for many years in the belief that it is the job which is affecting him, or a woman may suddenly decide she wants to change house because she becomes convinced that the neighbours have turned against her. (In general terms it is worth while encouraging a depressive *not* to make any important decisions during the active phase of his illness since his judgement is usually affected to a greater or lesser extent.)

Some depressives show a complete inability to make decisions when they are ill and they dither endlessly in their work and at home. Many are irritable: nothing seems right and nothing pleases. This may cause disturbances in interpersonal relationships and sometimes the patient turns away from company altogether and becomes solitary and asocial. Rudeness and tactlessness, often quite out of character, may cause embarrassment and offence to others.

Some depressive illnesses express themselves in strange ways. A respectable individual may commit an offence: for example, a patient known to us, a middle-aged woman who had developed a severe depression so insidiously that it had not been noticed, was caught stealing one meat-cube in a supermarket. She had absolutely no history of misdemeanours of this nature, and the "crime" was quite ludicrous. Unfortunately the manager of the shop wanted to press charges and it was only with some difficulty that he was persuaded not to. The woman could offer no explanation for her action and was overwhelmed with guilt feelings. Fortunately it became so obvious that she was ill that the authorities took the matter no further and the patient did extremely well with antidepressant treatment.

The Onset of Depressive Illness

Depressive conditions usually come on gradually, sometimes over a quite considerable period, even as much as a year or more. When the onset is so insidious, the illness may not be appreciated for what it is and medical advice will only be sought at a relatively late stage. In some instances, during the development of the illness the patient's life may be changed and, for example, his reduced efficiency at work may lead to his dismissal. When something like this occurs this effect of the illness is sometimes regarded as a cause. Some patients claim that their illness has come on suddenly, but even in these cases, careful history taking will often reveal that there has been a preceding period when they have been "off colour" in a non-specific way.

As already explained, some cases of depression are so disguised by physical symptoms that the patient undergoes all sorts of investigations before the nature of the illness becomes apparent. At other times, it is only when the person attempts or commits suicide that it is realized that a depressive illness has been present.

The Variability of the Depressive Picture

Text-books describe "typical" cases of depression, but in practice, cases are often quite uncharacteristic. The symptoms we have already described may or may not be present, may occur in varying combinations and may show any degree of severity. The picture will be further complicated by the fact that depression does not occur in a vacuum: it occurs in the setting of the individual's personality and the features of the personality are bound to affect the appearance of the illness, sometimes profoundly. Depression occurring in an obsessional middle-aged man may at times be difficult to recognize as the same illness as depression in a rather hare-brained, twenty-year-old girl.

On occasion the depression is so atypical that it is not possible to make a diagnosis from the actual appearance of the condition. Instead, the psychiatrist has to rely on factors such as the presence of a positive family history, a history of a previous attack of affective illness or even, in some cases, the response to antidepressant treatment which has been given on the basis of an informed hunch.

The Causation of Depressive Illness

Mood-swings are to be regarded as part of normal experience but depressive illness is a pathological occurrence. It follows a characteristic course and usually responds to antidepressant treatments. As yet we know relatively little about its actual causes, but some interesting facts can be mentioned.

It is likely that, in many cases, important hereditary factors are present. Though not invariable, a family history of affective disorders is relatively common in depressive illness. It is sometimes suggested that this indicates the effect of family influence rather than of hereditary factors, but there is evidence that a genetic influence is at work. For example, studies have been carried out on twin-pairs, one member of which suffers from affective illness, and it has been shown that the risk of the other twin developing a similar illness is much higher in identical pairs (where the genetic constitution is identical) than in non-identical pairs (where the genetic constitution is no more alike than in normal sibs). This appears to be true even where the twins have been raised apart since earliest life. As well as this, depressive illness often skips generations so that a patient's family history may relate to a grandparent or a cousin who could scarcely have had much direct influence on his upbringing.

The genetic factor, whatever its nature, apparently does not invariably lead to the development of the illness. It seems to provide some kind of predisposition to depression, but other factors are required to bring out the predisposition. Some of these may be constitutional in nature. For example, the illness, as we have seen, occurs more often in women than in men. (Part of this may be due to menstrual factors since many women experience marked mood-swings at the time of their menstrual periods.) In addition, it appears to occur rather more commonly in the stockily built individual (the "pyknic" physique) than in the person who is sparely built, and it also has some association with high blood pressure.

Such influences may add to the likelihood of an individual developing depressive illness. If, in addition, he possesses a cyclothymic type of personality (see p. 130) this likelihood will be increased. Sometimes the actual attack of depression appears to be precipitated by a traumatic event or an emotional disturbance (for example, a bereavement), but often there is no obvious precipitating factor. We have no good explanation for the recurrent nature of the illness except to say vaguely that some mechanism in the brain is at fault. (One tentative explanation which has been suggested is that depression is a kind of throw-back to a hibernating type of behaviour which was present in a distant non-human ancestor. This is no more than an interesting thought.)

The psychoanalytic explanation for depression postulates a partial arrest of libido at a very early stage of the child's development. In the early stage of infancy the child is totally dependent on the mother and gratification arises mainly from the ingestion of milk: this is the oral phase of development. If some traumatic event occurs at this time a certain amount of the primitive emotion will be bound down: this might occur, for example, if the child is separated from its mother and does not obtain adequate substitute care. This infant may then grow into an adult who has an excessive need for supplies of comfort and affection from others.

Emotional trauma in adult life may reawaken the primitive emotions: this is said to be especially true of situations where there is loss or threatened loss of the loved object. There is a desire to incorporate the loved object in order to prevent its being lost. Such a cannibalistic notion is acceptable to a very young child, but in the adult it is unacceptable and will cause severe feelings of guilt.

In our relationships with other people we have an image of them, a symbolic representation, within our own minds. When someone is very important to us that image naturally occupies a considerable niche and if we are separated from the person we have to learn to adapt to this new situation. The depressive individual finds it very difficult to accept the consequences of bereavement. His traumatic experience in childhood has left him with a tendency to ambivalence towards the loved object: he loves but he also hates and fears because he was deserted. Thus, when he is again deserted (as he sees it), he is angry and pleased at the same time and neither of these seems appropriate to a grief situation so he feels guilty on both accounts. In addition, in depression, the superego regresses to a harsh and primitive method of functioning and this adds to the individual's burden of guilt.

It should be said that this formulation of the aetiology of depression is conjectural. Many children undergo bereavement and do not become depressives, while many depressives have never suffered undue frustration in their early lives. The actual cause of depressive illness remains unclear.

The last point to make about the causation of depressive illness is that some cases of the condition are due to other illnesses, both psychiatric and physical. Typical depressive symptoms may be an early sign of schizophrenic illness or may appear in the course of a chronic obsessional neurosis. Depressive illness may arise following an attack of influenza or during an attack of jaundice and it is very common in elderly people suffering from hardening of the cerebral arteries. It is therefore always necessary to be aware that depression can be covering another condition so that the latter is not overlooked.

The Course of Depressive Illness

During the illness the mood will tend to sink until it reaches a nadir and then, because the condition is usually self-limiting, it will tend to start returning to normal again. This will happen even without treatment. Sometimes an attack will be relatively short-lived, lasting only a few days or weeks, but at other times it may be very prolonged and last up to several years. A small proportion do not clear up and this chronic illness can be very disabling.

One can always be optimistic about the prospects of recovery from an individual attack, especially with modern treatment, but the long-term prospect is much more difficult to assess since the illness does have a tendency to recur. Unfortunately it is often impossible to predict which patients will never have another attack. In general, the earlier the illness appears the more chance there is that it will occur again, and, of course, if a person has already had an episode of affective illness when one sees him this makes it all the more likely that he is suffering from a recurrent form of the condition and may be at greater risk for future episodes.

Never be tempted to give an opinion to a depressive or his relative about the possibility of a recurrence. It is good policy to concentrate on the current illness and to be optimistic about it. Depressives often tend to be worriers and if a man is told that his illness has a 50 : 50 chance of reappearing he may well spend much of his time worrying himself into a further attack. We have to be realistic about the situation in our own minds, but if the patient asks a question about the chance of the illness reappearing he usually wants reassurance rather than cold fact. If he is very persistent in his enquiry, arrange for him to talk the matter over with his general practitioner or psychiatrist.

Treatment

Even quite marked degrees of depression can be treated outside hospital nowadays, but if the illness is very severe or if there is a possibility of suicide the person must be admitted to hospital.

Depressive illness is usually an eminently treatable condition. In the mildest cases all the patient needs is reassurance and possibly mild sedation to help him relax and sleep better and the condition will rapidly cure itself. In more severe cases, one of the antidepressant drugs is often employed. These are not stimulants (like amphetamine), but are substances which raise the mood to a normal level and maintain it there till natural recovery occurs: usually there is a time-lag of 10 to 14 days before their effect becomes obvious and this has to be carefully explained to the patient, or else he will become discouraged and stop taking them.

The patient who is too severely depressed to respond to drugs may be given electroconvulsive therapy (E.C.T., electroplexy). This is usually a highly effective method of cutting short an attack of severe depression.

In E.C.T. an electric current is passed through the brain by means of a special apparatus. This treatment appears barbarous to many laymen and perhaps requires a brief word of explanation. In the early days of its use it was an unpleasant procedure because a by-product of the passage of the current was that the patient had an epileptic fit (hence electro-*convulsive* therapy). Nowadays the patient is given a short-acting general anaesthetic and a muscle-relaxant drug. When the current is passed he is quite unconscious of this and the only physical effect is a slight twitch of the muscles. Some patients have a degree of memory disturbance after a treatment but this is almost always transitory. A course of E.C.T. usually consists of between four and ten treatments. Nowadays fewer treatments are required because of the simultaneous use of anti-depressant drugs.

Sometimes tranquillizing drugs are required in addition to anti-depressant treatment when the patient is very tense and agitated. As you can see, the stress is largely on physical methods of treatment in the acute stage of the illness but other factors must not be neglected. As the illness resolves, the patient may be left with a considerable degree of anxiety, often partly due to worry about his illness. This will need at least reassurance and sometimes will necessitate the starting of a course of psychotherapy.

Where can the social worker help in the treatment of depression? In the great majority of cases recovery is going to take place and the person's life is only temporarily interrupted. Usually he will be able to take up where the illness made him leave off, both at work and in his personal relations, so his social problems may be relatively slight. Nevertheless, in a severe attack the patient will have to be in hospital, which invariably creates domestic problems. It may sometimes be necessary to reassure an employer that the condition is a temporary one and that recovery can be expected: many employers still become unnecessarily anxious about the possibility of an employee being permanently affected in some way. If the patient, because of his illness, has made a rash decision such as throwing up his work, he may require practical guidance to help obtain other employment. During the process of recovery, self-confidence may take some time to reappear and feelings of inadequacy may persist unduly. This may interfere with the patient's ability to work efficiently and friendly encouragement from the social worker is likely to help him greatly.

The outpatient depressive may need some social support, and if there are any factors in the environment which are detrimental to his morale it may be necessary to deal with these: for example, housing may be unsuitable or there may be debts, etc. It may be very reassuring to the individual to know that his relatives and dependants are being helped while he is ill.

Finally, the social worker should note any fluctuations in the person's mood-state and any ideas of suicide which may be expressed. These observations should be communicated immediately to the psychiatrist: they may not indicate very much in the majority of instances, but suicide is the greatest danger in depressive illness and its possibility should never be ignored.

Mania

In many ways this condition can be regarded as the opposite side of the coin from depression and in a certain proportion of cases mania and depression will occur alternately in the same individual. It is said that the same intra-psychic conflicts occur in mania as in depression (see pp. 211 ff), but that the manic patient denies these in a massive fashion. The depressive mechanisms are repressed (the so-called "manic defence") and the patient swings to the opposite mood-extreme, becoming over-elated. Whatever the psychopathology of the process, hereditary and constitutional factors appear to be as important as in depressive illness.

Symptoms of Mania

The central feature is the mood of elation which is so intense and so sustained that it cannot be regarded as appropriate to the circumstances. Many lay people find it difficult to accept that mania can be an illness because the patient usually claims to feel exceptionally well and he is often patently extremely cheerful. However, there are additional features which present a less happy picture.

The manic shows marked over-confidence and a profound loss of self-criticism which may amount to total lack of insight into his own abnormal behaviour. He is over-active and this annoys others more than himself: he will cheerfully rise at 3 a.m. and start making noisy preparations to begin the day, oblivious to the disturbance he is creating. His over-activity is usually inconsistent and he rarely achieves anything. He talks incessantly, darting rapidly from one topic to another. His thoughts are speeded up and show a marked tendency to take flight (the phenomenon is called "flight of ideas").

Thinking and speech are governed by his distractibility and are influenced by casual noises in the environment, punning, rhymes and so on. There is often an air of hilarity about his manner and his conversation which can readily infect the onlooker: it is said that one of the diagnostic features in mania is that the other person cannot help laughing with (as opposed to laughing *at*) the patient. However, the patient is not invariably happy. Sometimes his thoughts are so accelerated that he becomes intolerant of ordinary mortals who seem unable to keep up with him, and he may show much irritability and at times he may have outbursts of violent temper and behaviour. Some manic patients become very tense and anxious and some show a strange admixture of manic and depressive symptoms.

The Onset of Mania

This is often a good deal more rapid than in depression and may sometimes be quite sudden. In some cases mania occurs when a depressive illness has apparently recovered but the mood has "overshot" normality and continued to swing upwards.

A manic rarely comes to a doctor spontaneously asking for treatment: the doctor is usually brought to the patient by despairing relatives who cannot understand the person's altered behaviour. Particularly if the condition comes on gradually, the relatives may well not understand that it is an illness and may show extraordinary tolerance of the individual's increasingly tactless, noisy behaviour, may forgive his insults and may overlook his childish pranks. But even these abnormalities of behaviour will come to be overshadowed by the development of grandiose delusions, violent outbursts or sexual promiscuity. It is often only then that it becomes obvious that the person is very unwell.

The Course of the Manic Illness

Most cases of mania are, just as with depression, self-limiting. It is a good deal less common than depression (and some authorities believe that it is becoming rarer with the passage of time for some reason), but it is possible that many mild cases go unrecognized because an illness characterized by good spirits and increased drive and optimism is unlikely to be thought of as pathological. Like depression, the illness shows a tendency to increase to a peak, then to start waning. The length of an individual attack varies widely from individual to individual and there is a decided trend in some cases towards chronicity.

Hypomania

Some cases never develop the extreme symptoms of the condition and the illness is then known as hypomania: these patients will tend to show some over-activity and distractibility, but usually do not become grossly deluded. Nevertheless, lack of insight and a degree of recklessness combined with the other none-too-noticeable features of the illness may enable the patient to do all sorts of irresponsible things before his relatives realize what is happening. When this occurs, the effects may be more devastating from a social viewpoint than with mania because it will be difficult to persuade creditors and others that the person was not responsible for his actions.

Treatment of Mania

A great difficulty often arises in persuading the patient to accept treatment. It is usually wise to bring the patient into hospital to minimize the possible consequences of his abnormal behaviour and in severe cases he may have to be compelled to enter hospital if he refuses to co-operate. In milder cases where compulsion is inappropriate the utmost powers of persuasion may be needed to induce the person to come to hospital and to remain once he is there.

Treatment usually takes the form of administration of powerful tranquillizing and sedative drugs to bring the mood-state back to normal. In severe cases, electroconvulsive therapy may be required. Most cases respond well but the drugs may have to be continued for long periods. Unfortunately if the illness flares up this is often the signal for the patient to stop taking the treatment because he feels too well to require it.

Occasionally mania or hypomania becomes very chronic and

defies treatment. In these cases the picture is often that of a persistently over-active, querulous, paranoid individual with a noisy sense of humour, no tact and a habit of behaving unpredictably. As is well known, not by any means all of such people are in hospital.

The Social Worker's Contribution to Treatment

Treatment for the patient is mostly by physical means in the early stages of the illness, but he requires help and encouragement to enable him to accept treatment. A direct approach often makes him angry and stubborn, but a friendly attitude on the part of the doctor and social worker will often persuade him to be cooperative.

But even more important at this stage of the disorder is the social worker's role in helping the family and dependants. By the time the patient reaches medical attention his family may be destitute because he has run up debts, quarrelled with his employers, indulged in extramarital adventures and so on. The family is often in a state of utter bewilderment and needs a great deal of explanation and support (including moral support to withstand the patient's demands that he should be taken out of hospital because he is perfectly well). Practical help and advice will often also be necessary.

In the milder cases of hypomania the patient will usually have little difficulty in returning to his normal life, but after a really severe illness he may need a great deal of assistance to enable him to pick up the threads again, particularly if he has lost his job, perhaps strained his marital relations and antagonized his friends. During the period of return to normality there is always a danger of depression developing and a close watch should be kept for signs of this happening.

B. SCHIZOPHRENIA

The term "Schizophrenia" covers a group of severe mental illnesses which are not caused by any known form of brain damage but which show as a characteristic feature a very marked tendency to produce destruction and disintegration of the personality. In the majority of cases this disintegration is progressive and would result in permanent impairment of the mental state unless the patient received treatment. There is no true intellectual deterioration (though thinking may show a tendency to get into a marked rut) and if a patient recovers he may do so fully, which suggests that there is not necessarily a permanently destructive process at work.

The manifestations of schizophrenia are legion, so much so that some psychiatrists talk about "The Schizophrenias" implying that there are a number of related but distinct illnesses. Against this idea to some extent is the observation that the picture often changes from one form of the condition to another in the same individual.

At one time schizophrenia was known as Dementia Praecox because it was considered to be a form of intellectual deterioration (dementia) and appeared to affect only young people (praecox is basically the same word as precocious). Its present name was substituted when it became obvious that it was not a dementing process and that it not infrequently affected older people. Schizophrenia literally means "split mind" and nowadays, apart from its real meaning, the term tends to be misused in two ways: it is sometimes employed when the person means "in two minds" in the sense of being indecisive and sometimes when describing an individual with a "Jekyll and Hyde" type of personality. Neither of these usages represents the situation in schizophrenia in which the personality not only splits; it shatters and disintegrates into a mass of poorly co-operating components. In particular there is a marked degree of dissociation between thought and emotion.

As yet we cannot diagnose schizophrenia in an objective way. Often the illness presents a characteristic picture, but when we analyse its features item by item we find that most of them can be found at some time or another in conditions other than schizophrenia. When asked to say how they diagnose the illness many psychiatrists will say that they use the criterion that it "cannot be understood". This may seem a strange way to make a diagnosis, but the implication is that, after exhaustive investigations, no understandable connection can be discerned between the symptoms of the illness and what has gone before in the patient's personality, his intellectual processes and his emotional experiences. Some psychiatrists would say more pithily that, if at the end of an interview with a patient they know that one or other of them is mentally ill, but they are not sure which, then the diagnosis is schizophrenia! This may appear facetious, but in fact one of the striking features of the illness is that the patient is emotionally aloof and this often creates an atmosphere of oddness and apartness in the interview situation which is difficult to pinpoint and sometimes causes the interviewer to think that he is losing his grip. One can only learn this experience by dealing with schizophrenics and, if the truth be told, one can only really learn about schizophrenia by coming in contact with a series of cases which display the features of the illness.

Symptoms of Schizophrenia

In schizophrenia there is profound disruption of ego-function with severe distortion of the patient's concept of self. He loses contact with reality to a greater or lesser extent and tends to withdraw into his own fantasy world. The relationship between himself and the outside world is impaired and he may lose the ability to experience emotional rapport with other human beings. Often these phenomena produce feelings of great perplexity in the patient but they occur in a setting of clear consciousness and the interruption of mental function is not brought about by confusion.

It is customary to consider the numerous symptoms of schizophrenia according to the particular aspects of psychic functioning which are affected. We shall mention briefly the manifestations of the illness under six headings: disorders of thought, emotion and volition, psychomotor symptoms, hallucinations and delusions.

1. *Disorders of thought.* Thinking may be affected in a variety of ways. For example, the schizophrenic finds difficulty in thinking in abstract terms. His responses to questions often appear strange because they concentrate on the concrete aspects of a subject. This is readily shown by asking him to explain the meaning of a proverb such as "People in glass houses should not throw stones". The

patient's reply is likely to be to the effect that people who live in glass houses who throw stones will break their windows: he concentrates on the literal rather than on the proverbial meaning. In addition he often displays Overinclusive Thinking: being unable to see the wood for the trees, his thinking and conversation on a particular subject are apt to drag in all sorts of irrelevancies.

The phenomenon of thought-blocking is very characteristic: here the patient experiences a cessation of his thoughts and for a short time the mind is completely blank. This is more than just a period of "wool-gathering" and the sensation is usually very disturbing to the patient. It may come to be associated with the delusion that thoughts are being stolen from his head. Sometimes when his thoughts appear alien and strange he may get the opposite delusion and believe that he is having thoughts forced into his head.

The conversation is frequently odd and stilted. The syntax may be disturbed and sometimes neologisms are sprinkled through the patient's speech: these are words which he himself has created. (Compare Lewis Carroll's "Twas brillig and the slithey toves".) Occasionally the patient will come to speak a gobbledygook jargon of his own which is utterly incomprehensible.

2. *Disorders of emotion.* Particularly at the beginning of the illness almost any emotional change may be seen. Anxiety and perplexity are common and sometimes a very typical manic-depressive reaction occurs. As the illness develops the emotions become progressively flatter so that the person comes to show little reaction to events, but this flattening may sometimes be interrupted by outbursts of severe and primitive affect such as rage, fear or hilarity. Emotional expression becomes awkward and incongruity of affect is common, the patient weeping when he is told something amusing or giggling when he learns some sad news! Splitting of affect may occur: here, thinking and emotion become quite detached from each other.

3. *Disorders of volition.* Initiative is often profoundly diminished so that the patient just sits around and neglects his work and duties.

He may talk a great deal about what he intends to do, but the intention is rarely translated into action. Sometimes he displays negativism, in which state he either refuses absolutely to do what he is asked or else does the exact opposite.

4. *Psychomotor symptoms*. Various types of block may develop between intention and the action to carry out that intention and abnormalities of behaviour and movement known as catatonic symptoms arise. The patient may slow up to the point where he remains motionless for long periods or he may even become stuporose. At other times he may have outbursts of violent over-activity sometimes associated with primitive destructiveness and aggressiveness. (Violence in schizophrenia is very much the exception but it never pays to take chances with a disturbed catatonic schizophrenic.)

5. *Hallucinatory symptoms*. An hallucination is a sensory perception which occurs in the absence of an external stimulus. The commonest hallucinations in schizophrenia are auditory: the patient may say that he hears noises such as humming or buzzing or he may hear voices. Sometimes these voices will tell him to do things; occasionally they say pleasant things to him, but more usually they are abusive and frightening. He may think that he hears his thoughts being spoken aloud and this will lead him to believe that other people can appreciate what he is thinking.

Other hallucinations which may occur include sensations of taste or smell (usually unpleasant), tingling feelings which are interpreted as electric shocks, and sensations in the genital regions which cause the person to think that he or she is being interfered with sexually: great embarrassment may be caused if they accuse some innocent bystander of assault. Visual hallucinations are uncommon.

Sometimes the patient suffers from illusions rather than hallucinations. In this case he does not imagine the stimulus, but he misinterprets it just as a child frightened by shadows might imagine they were people out to harm him.

6. *Delusions*. A delusion is an over-valued belief which is obviously false to other people but to which the individual clings unreasonably.

Delusions are a form of thought-disorder and they occur very frequently in schizophrenia. Characteristically there is a Primary Delusion which suddenly presents itself to the patient's consciousness like an inspiration, then this is followed by numerous secondary delusional beliefs, many of which are attempts by the individual to explain his puzzling and frightening new experiences. For example, a man may develop the belief that he is heir to a vast fortune and then has to explain that his lack of ready money is due to the fact that a gang of people are conspiring against him to deny him his inheritance. Not infrequently delusions take on a decidedly persecutory tinge. Sometimes they become extremely grandiose and often there is a strong element of religiosity. (In one hospital ward there were once two patients who thought that they were Christ: one of them confided to a doctor that he thought the other patient should be removed because he was an impostor.)

The Schizophrenic Illness

Having listed a large number of schizophrenic symptoms it should be said that modern treatment should prevent many of them from appearing. Many of the descriptions of schizophrenia in text-books are of chronic cases whose symptoms have been aggravated by years of institutionalization. It is the psychiatrist's pipe-dream to be able to identify schizophrenia before any serious manifestations occur, but so far this remains largely wishful thinking. The illness can certainly be treated, but though the outlook is not exceptionally good for the individual patient there should never be undue delay in starting treatment.

While any combination of schizophrenic symptoms may occur, in practice it is usually possible to consign a case to one of four main categories. These are not exclusive and in the course of time or as the result of treatment a patient may change from one type of illness to another. If the condition becomes chronic the picture consists of a complex mixture of positive symptoms such as delusions and hallucinations and negative symptoms such as lack of emotional drive, emotional flatness and poverty of thought. The four types of schizophrenia are Simple, Hebephrenic, Paranoid and Catatonic.

1. *Simple schizophrenia.* This type is mostly characterized by negative symptoms. The most noticeable of these is the shallowness of the emotional response, which may range from some degree of indifference to the most gross callousness. There is usually a marked absence of drive, and thought disorder (particularly poverty of ideas and thought-blocking) is often present. Insight is often completely lacking so the individual is usually not much disturbed by his condition and often feels little need to seek medical treatment.

The onset of simple schizophrenia is usually insidious and the illness often progresses very gradually. This means that it is often not recognized for a considerable time and by the time it is it will have taken firm root. Sometimes it comes to a halt and the person is able to make some form of precarious adjustment, but more often he drifts away from family, friends and work and gradually drops down the social scale. Personality, interpersonal relationships and occupational ability suffer. Some simple schizophrenics become incompetently criminal, others are readily persuaded to take to drugs. Many just become drifters and vagrants: many tramps and doss-house inmates are simple schizophrenics and in the women prostitution is common.

Sometimes the appearance closely resembles that of the schizoid personality (see p. 131), but the crucial difference is that the simple schizophrenic has undergone a profound change of personality, usually in the late teens or early twenties. Occasionally the change is not insidious and the typical picture of simple schizophrenia may appear following an acute illness. Whatever the mode of onset, the outlook in this illness is extremely poor.

2. *Hebephrenic schizophrenia.* In this type of illness thought-disorder and emotional disturbances are the most prominent features. This is the commonest form of schizophrenia in young people and its appearances are extremely varied. The thought disorder may vary from mild vagueness to the most profound disorganization of thinking. At first, dreaminess and inability to concentrate are common but outbursts of inappropriate and sometimes violent emotion often occur and the patient frequently complains of depression.

The onset may be sudden but is often gradual and may be mistaken for neurosis or depression. In young people it may be taken for adolescent turmoil and sometimes it is thought that the patient is deliberately playing the fool, because the behaviour may be flippant and buffoonish. As the illness progresses a rather empty silliness of manner is frequent, although sometimes the individual becomes portentous and the apparent profundity of his meaningless remarks are often sufficiently impressive-sounding to fool people for a time. The conversation and behaviour develop an odd, bizarre quality: delusions may become florid and hallucinations often become persistent. Hebephrenic schizophrenia tends to be progressive and to have a poor outcome.

3. *Paranoid schizophrenia.* Here the outstanding features are delusions and hallucinations, but in many cases the personality of the patient does not deteriorate nearly so markedly as in the other forms. Sometimes indeed the personality remains relatively intact and the patient appears able to dissociate his illness from his normal sphere of mental activity. When this happens he may be able to remain in society and function at a moderately effective level: no one may realize that he is suffering from an illness but he is often recognized as being somewhat eccentric.

The word "paranoid" really means "delusional", but is used by many people to imply delusions of persecution: thus the term "paranoid delusion" has come to be virtually synonymous with persecutory delusion. Often the paranoid schizophrenic's delusions do have a persecutory content and as well as this they may be extremely grandiose. At times the patient may experience the most intense waves of emotion which may take the form of elation, bliss, ecstasy or rage: these may be interpreted by him as evidence of some form of religious visitation.

Paranoid schizophrenia is an illness which most typically affects the middle-aged or even elderly person (it can occur right into extreme old age). It often seems to occur in individuals who are predisposed to the extent that their previous personality was odd and it is excessively common in the unmarried and divorced (but not in the widowed). It tends to be a very chronic condition: the outlook is good to the extent that the personality is relatively well retained, but the delusional system often proves very resistant to treatment.

4. *Catatonic schizophrenia.* This illness frequently begins much more suddenly than the others and usually occurs in adolescence or young adulthood. Its onset is dominated by psychomotor symptoms such as immobility, posturing and stupor, sometimes alternating with outbursts of frenzied over-activity and violence. Behaviour and speech are stiff and stereotyped and the patient may display phenomena such as negativism or automatic obedience.

Despite the profound disturbance of behaviour and the frequently bizarre appearance of the patient this form of the illness more often shows a tendency to remit and to respond to treatment. Part of this responsiveness may be due to the rapidity of onset of the condition which allows treatment to start at a relatively early stage.

The Onset of Schizophrenia

This has been described already for each individual type of schizophrenia: in general it is an illness of gradual onset and at first the symptoms are quite non-specific. When the onset is *very* sudden one should keep in mind the possibility of the illness being due to the effects of drugs because substances such as amphetamine, L.S.D. and mescaline sometimes produce appearances quite indistinguishable from schizophrenia.

Schizophrenia proper is mostly an illness of young people which starts to be common after puberty and has passed its peak incidence by the age of 30. Because of its frequently progressive and destructive nature, schizophrenia is not diagnosed lightly, but whenever the illness is suspected in someone, that person must be persuaded to accept a period of observation till the diagnosis is clinched one way or the other. Thereafter, if schizophrenia is present, treatment should be started as soon as possible.

The Previous Personality of the Schizophrenic

As with many psychiatric illnesses, we see the schizophrenic once his illness has begun to have effects on his personality so it is difficult to be too dogmatic about the characteristics of his premorbid character. However, there seems little doubt that a considerable proportion (perhaps as many as half) of schizophrenics show marked abnormalities before their illness. The characteristic features they display are those of being excessively quiet, shy and withdrawn. They have a poor ability to demonstrate emotion and they tend to be asocial. These are features of the "schizoid" personality which is not uncommonly found in the general population. Most schizoid individuals never develop schizophrenia, but they do have a somewhat excessive liability to develop the condition, and schizoid personalities are found fairly frequently amongst the relatives of schizophrenics.

Sometimes a simple schizophrenic illness ceases to advance before it has affected the individual profoundly and the picture which results may closely resemble the schizoid state. Also, some schizophrenics who have received treatment lose their most florid symptoms, but continue to have mild features which again resemble those of the schizoid personality.

It should be remembered that approximately half of the cases of schizophrenia arise in people whose previous personality was apparently normal.

Predisposing Factors in Schizophrenia

Schizophrenia appears to occur in all human cultures and it affects both sexes equally. It occurs more frequently in those at the bottom of the socio-economic scale than in those higher up, but this mostly seems to indicate that schizophrenia causes people to drift downwards in society and to accumulate amongst the poor earners. It is similarly found to excess among those who live alone or who live solitary lives in doss-houses, probably for the same reason. There is no evidence that the illness is caused by a particular way of life.

There is probably an important hereditary factor in schizophrenia and a positive family history is commonly found. The nature of the hereditary element is unknown but its significance appears to be confirmed by twin studies. The closer a person's degree of blood-relationship is to a schizophrenic the greater is the risk of his developing a similar illness. For example, it is said that the risk of a member of the general population developing schizophrenia at some time during his life is about 0·5 to 0·8 per cent: for the sib of a schizophrenic the risk is approximately 10 per cent.

Constitutional factors are involved and there is some connection between the asthenic body-build (the physique with a tendency to be skinny and droopy) and a tendency to develop schizophrenia. However, it must be remembered that many schizophrenics are adolescents who often tend to be rather droopy at this age in any case.

The illness itself may have an effect on appearance and many schizophrenics undergoing treatment put on a good deal of weight. But there are other well-known associated physical abnormalities such as low blood-pressure, cold blue extremities and greasy skin and it can be shown that in many schizophrenics the biochemical response to stress differs from normal. However, none of these phenomena have ever been shown to be exclusive to schizophrenia. There is one small group of patients who suffer from a schizophrenia-like condition called Periodic Catatonia and their symptoms are due to an intermittent accumulation of nitrogen in the body. This can be successfully treated by giving thyroid hormone in large doses and this clears out the excess of nitrogenous substances. Unfortunately, when this treatment is tried in true schizophrenia very little beneficial effect is obtained.

Many people believe that schizophrenia is caused by some, as yet unknown, biochemical abnormality: this abnormality could arise within the brain itself or could be the result of toxic substances produced in another part of the body and reaching the brain by way of the blood-stream. Numerous investigations on this topic are now being carried out but so far no definite proof has emerged. Some weight has been lent to the biochemical theory by the fact that states which resemble schizophrenia in some ways can be produced temporarily by chemical substances such as mescaline and lysergic acid diethylamide (L.S.D.).

Schizophrenia often begins in the absence of any obvious precipitating factor and even where there seems to have been some form of stress this is sometimes found to be a result of the illness rather than a cause of it. To take an example, the relative of a schizophrenic may say that the patient's illness began as a result of his losing his job. When the story is gone into carefully it sometimes transpires that what has actually happened is that the illness has been coming on slowly, causing a gradual change in the man's behaviour and a consequent falling-off in his work performance. His superiors have not realized that this drop in efficiency has been brought about by illness and have dismissed him. It is only afterwards, in many cases, that the illness becomes obvious.

Occasionally schizophrenia begins after a physical illness but, on the other hand, it has sometimes been reported that a schizophrenic can improve temporarily during the course of another illness. A small number of schizophrenic illnesses begin soon after childbirth (puerperal schizophrenia). In older people particularly, a schizophrenic illness often appears to have its onset after the death of a close relative. A not uncommon story is of two elderly spinster sisters living together and when one dies the other develops strange and bizarre symptoms. Again, care must be taken not to assume too quickly that the schizophrenia was caused by the bereavement. It may be that the survivor has always been eccentric and has been cared for by the deceased relative whose death leaves the patient observably incapable of looking after herself.

Significant Events in Early Life

A great deal of theoretical discussion has taken place about the influence of the family and particularly of the mother in predisposing some children to schizophrenia, but we have very little apart from anecdotal information on this topic. It has been suggested by a number of workers that schizophrenics are particularly likely to have suffered from parental deprivation or the effects of a broken home, but for every study which reports this finding there is one which has found no evidence to support the theory. Even if a history of broken home were found to be especially common, this would not necessarily tell us very much about the genesis of the illness: many parents of schizophrenics who are not themselves suffering from the illness are nevertheless odd and difficult people, often with schizoid traits, and it would not be surprising, in view of their inability to sustain personal relationships, to find that their marriages readily broke down.

It has been proposed at various times that a certain type of mother is likely to create schizophrenia in the child by her behaviour towards it. Typically, this mother is unable to show spontaneous affection and is aloof and unresponsive to the child's needs. She is unable to form adequate emotional bonds with the infant and she may show great ambivalence towards him. This ambivalence may express itself in "Double Bind" situations where the parent gives the child impossibly contradictory commands: a mild example (which certainly crops up also in non-schizophrenic households) would be, "Mummy wants you to enjoy yourself but don't get yourself untidy." A more damaging instance is the situation where mother encourages the child almost in a seductive way to show love, then angrily rejects the child's affection, causing him much bewilderment. The child who is consistently thwarted in this way will never learn the basic rules of forming interpersonal relationships and he may develop a tendency to become too introspective and withdrawn from reality.

Some people go so far as to assert that the schizophrenic is less disturbed than his parent: that the parent has a stronger personality and retains some grip on sanity whereas the affected child breaks down and retreats into illness to escape the intolerable strain of living with such a parent. There is no adequate proof for this view and it begs such questions as why it is that only a proportion of children in an abnormal family develop this illness while the others escape: it also fails to explain the large number of schizophrenics who develop their illness after an apparently normal upbringing and early life. All in all, the malignant effect of mother's behaviour seems to have been overrated and schizophrenia seems just as likely to arise in a family where father is abnormal in some way, or often in a family where neither parent is abnormal.

The widest consensus of opinion nowadays seems to be that the various factors we have just mentioned may have some part to play, but without the underlying constitutional predisposition the illness cannot appear.

Psychoanalytic formulation. It is fairly widely agreed that there is no psychodynamic theory which provides a satisfactory explanation for the illness. Many of the symptoms of schizophrenia represent a profound degree of regression and it has been suggested that, as the Ego disintegrates, we begin to see the mechanisms of the Id exposed. Thought and emotion become primitive and the individual withdraws into himself, unable to maintain relationships with objects and people outside himself. Many schizophrenic manifestations are interpreted as the organism's desperate attempt to reconstruct order out of chaotic material.

Unfortunately, none of this explains schizophrenia: it only describes graphically what appears to be happening. To date even the most sophisticated psychological, social or biochemical theory has done no more than this.

The Treatment of Schizophrenia

Schizophrenia is an immense medico-social problem and the chronicity of the condition makes the problem even greater. Once the illness has occurred, in the great majority of cases it remains with the patient. If you catch a cold it stays with you for a few days and after that you are no longer a case of the cold. The person who develops schizophrenia at the age of twenty may well be a case of schizophrenia twenty years later. Even with treatment, there is a huge accumulation of cases and this is why schizophrenics have always formed such a high proportion of the psychiatric inpatient total. Some schizophrenics are never seen by a doctor. Usually these are the ones who just quietly develop into drifters, vagrants or prostitutes, or else they are paranoid schizophrenics who, though disturbed, just manage to keep a hold on their everyday lives. Otherwise most schizophrenics become sufficiently ill to require medical attention.

Until comparatively recently treatment for schizophrenics

largely consisted of admission to mental hospital and thereafter nursing and custodial care: under these conditions some patients recovered but the majority became chronic inmates and, as already explained, became hopelessly institutionalized. Nowadays even if the patient often has to be admitted to hospital the approach is entirely different. He will usually receive drugs (and sometimes electroconvulsive therapy) which control his disturbed behaviour and calm his mind so that he can remain in touch with his surroundings. The hospital environment should be designed to encourage him to maintain contact with reality and to prevent his withdrawing into himself. Every attempt is made to keep him in touch with his relatives and his everyday environment and the primary aim of treatment is to ensure his early discharge from hospital and his rehabilitation in the community.

Drug treatment in schizophrenia is ameliorative; that is to say, it controls symptoms but rarely seems to cure the illness. It is most effective when started early, but if it is discontinued the symptoms will usually begin to advance again. Nowadays we can often expect very good results from the use of powerful tranquillizers, but even a successful result from drug therapy is only a beginning. Once improvement begins the patient requires much help and support and other forms of treatment. Personal contact with nurses, doctors, social workers and other patients is very important and the patient should never be allowed to become detached and isolated. Active occupation should be provided and efforts made to ensure that this is not repetitive and tedious lest the patient gets into a rut. Indeed, in some mild cases, close human contact and the stimulating effect of a well-organized hospital milieu may be all that is required to initiate recovery.

The co-operation of the family must be enlisted, but this may not always be easy, particularly when some of its members are themselves disturbed. The relatives should be encouraged to visit the patient in hospital and he should start to spend short periods at home as soon as he is able to. Good communication is of the essence in the treatment situation and relatives should feel free to contact a member of the therapeutic team whenever the need arises, and the doctor or social worker should always be ready to listen and to provide appropriate help. The psychiatrist with a large number of patients on his case-load will depend very considerably on the social worker in this type of situation.

When the patient is reaching the stage when leaving hospital is imminent he will probably require help with employment. He may or may not be able to take up his previous work and he may or may not have insight into the particular problems caused by his illness. (Sometimes there is an inverse relationship between intelligence and the ability to resume the previous occupation: a highly skilled professional man who has made a good recovery from schizophrenia but whose ethical sense has been somewhat blunted by the illness may have much more difficulty in coping with his particular type of work than the unintelligent and unskilled man with an equally severe condition whose resulting personality deficits may be scarcely noticeable.)

It cannot be denied that the early discharge of schizophrenic patients causes many problems. The patient may no longer be able to maintain his family at a reasonable economic level and sometimes he may become an economic liability. His behaviour may not be completely normal and there may even be outbursts of very disturbed behaviour at times which may cause many tensions in the home. Perhaps worst of all, the family has to realize that this situation may continue for the rest of the individual's life. In view of the great burdens put upon the family and the community, social workers may be called upon to provide a good deal of practical help and moral support for both the patient and the family.

Many schizophrenics, despite strenuous efforts to prevent it happening, become detached from their families and backgrounds and they require a great deal of help with accommodation and a lot of supportive supervision. In some parts of the country there are half-way houses and hostels for the discharged schizophrenic, but in many places there is no satisfactory service for the care of the homeless schizophrenic ex-patient. Even those who do have a home and relatives have to be considered as individual cases and it would obviously be of little use sending a schizophrenic back to a home which is utterly disorganized as a result of the relatives also being disturbed. Some patients, on the other hand, find it overwhelming when they try to return to the normal emotional relationships of home and these cases sometimes cope better in well-supervised lodgings or a hostel. Ideally there should be a concerted plan of action for each patient when he is discharged, but too often lack of facilities prevents this from happening.

Frequently, early discharge leads to great difficulties for the patient and his relatives which results in his early readmission. It has been said rather cynically that the hospital "open door" policy has become the "revolving door" policy. Such comment may be intended as a condemnation of our inadequate follow-up methods, but it may equally be that close supervision by competent social workers ensures that schizophrenics are returned for hospital treatment at an earlier stage because an incipient relapse is recognized almost immediately. It is certainly not wrong to try to prevent the patient from becoming an institutionalized "vegetable". One very potent reason for repeated readmission is that many patients fail to take their drugs regularly, partly through lack of drive and persistence and partly because of negative feelings engendered by their illness. In many cases adequate supervision could ensure that the medicines were being taken and this would reduce the breakdown rate. Here, as in every other aspect of the problem of the discharged schizophrenic, the observant and interested social worker may be able to play a significant part in the prevention of relapse.

Puerperal Psychosis

Many women suffer from a short period of "the blues" just after the birth of a child and this is so common as to be normal. The rather inadequate woman or the woman with a previous history of neurotic disorder may have a flare-up of psychoneurotic symptoms, often because she is afraid that she will be unable to cope with the infant. This type of anxiety usually responds to reassurance, sedation and, if necessary, psychotherapy.

In the days before antibiotic drugs were available, psychotic disturbances commonly followed childbirth, most of them being delirious illnesses caused by severe infections. This kind of disorder is now largely preventable, but functional psychotic disturbances still occur in the period following childbirth, the Puerperium. At one time it was thought that these functional puerperal psychoses had a peculiar form and a course which differed from those of other functional psychoses. Nowadays it is recognized that the puerperium is simply a period of increased risk for psychiatric illness, probably because of all the complex hormonal and emotional changes which occur at this time, and the puerperal psychoses themselves appear to be similar in content and in their response to treatment to comparable conditions arising at other periods of life. Some show a mixture of affective and schizophrenic symptoms, but most of them are typically manic-depressive or schizophrenic, though in a number of cases the appearances are temporarily complicated by mild delirious features.

The possible effects of a puerperal disturbance on the new-born infant must never be overlooked. If the illness is severe the mother will be patently unable to look after the child and the family or various social organizations will usually rally round while she is receiving treatment. On the other hand, the less dramatic forms of puerperal illness may go almost unnoticed and while they last the mother's ability to give care and affection is often seriously diminished. If, as sometimes happens, this situation continues for a long time the infant may suffer a considerable degree of emotional deprivation. The social worker should be aware of the possibility and preventability of this occurrence.

CHAPTER 10

Psychiatric Conditions due to Old Age and to Organic Causes

A. PSYCHIATRIC ILLNESS OF OLD AGE

When an old person becomes mentally ill it is natural to assume that this is evidence of deterioration due to senility and that there is very little that we can usefully do about the situation. However, this is far from necessarily being the case: it is by no means inevitable that an old person with a psychiatric disorder should continue to go downhill until he dies. There are various types of mental illness in old age and some of them are associated with a remarkably good recovery rate.

In the majority of old people deterioration of body and mind occur at about the same pace and if they enjoy good health the "winding-down" process will usually be sufficiently slow to ensure that they remain alert and useful members of society to the end. The greater proportion of old people do not become mentally deranged, although it can be shown that it is normal for them to undergo a progressive diminution of certain aspects of their intellectual capacity.

Human beings reach an intellectual peak in their early twenties and thereafter they undergo a gradual decline in abilities such as abstract thinking, problem solving and efficiency of memorization. By the time the fifties and sixties are reached the capacity for original thought has usually diminished greatly (though some exceptional old people retain this ability to an extremely advanced age), but this is to a large extent balanced by an increase in experience, maturity of judgement, and more stable, more highly directed emotional drive. These compensating factors can remain effective for many years in a well-balanced old person.

Undoubtedly most old people become less and less flexible in their attitudes with the passage of time. They compensate for their loss of adaptability by having a set formula for each situation and by avoiding new situations wherever possible. Since an old person tends in any case to become less mobile and his life rather restricted this formula usually works quite well, but obviously they must be vulnerable to any sudden change which is thrust upon them. For example, the elderly lady who uproots herself from her long-accustomed background to go to live with relatives or in an old folk's home may be quite unable to adapt to the new routines and may become peevish and irritable or even confused at times.

Memory is usually affected to a greater or lesser extent in old people. Again they minimize this by sticking closely to a routine so that everything is in its place and everything is done by rote. An old person's fussiness may sometimes be annoying, but it does serve a useful purpose in this way. Usually it is recent memory which is most affected and memories of the distant past are often unimpaired: in fact they sometimes appear to be enhanced. As a result the old person may find it easier to remember what happened fifty years ago than something that happened yesterday. They may spend long periods thinking and talking about events which took place in their youthful years: this is interesting the first time it is recounted, but it can become intensely irritating when it is repeated word for word on innumerable occasions.

Old people often annoy younger people because they are slow, they dwell a great deal in the past and they are apt to grumble about everything new or strange. Fortunately, the greater number of old folk are able to fend for themselves; but as medical care becomes progressively more effective more people live to be elderly and the number of disabled old people rises. As society becomes more mobile and as people find more things to occupy their attention, fewer young people are likely to want to take on the care of an aged relative: in any case, mobility of existence is likely to prove most uncongenial to the elderly.

The Pattern of Psychiatric Illness in Old People

We know comparatively little about the patterns of psychiatric illness among old people in the general community, but we do know that it is probably very common. Almost a sixth of our population is now of pensionable age: what proportion of these is suffering from mental disorders? It has been suggested by Roth and Kay (1962),* as the result of a community survey they carried out in Newcastle upon Tyne, that almost one-third of old people living at home suffer from some degree of psychiatric disturbance. What is particularly surprising about the findings in this study is that some two-thirds of these disturbed old people appeared to have various kinds of psychoneurotic illness and it is standard psychiatric teaching that such conditions are rarely found beyond middle age. Presumably psychiatrists have remained ignorant about psychoneuroses of old age because they usually do not provide sufficient cause for admission to hospital. Nevertheless, these old people function considerably less effectively than they otherwise might.

Most of the severe forms of mental illness are also present in the general population. In fact, there are probably more highly disturbed aged people outside hospital than inside. The pattern of psychotic illness in the elderly is influenced to some extent by the difference in mortality rates between the two sexes. In general, women live considerably longer than men, and men are more likely to suffer from strokes due to disease of the cerebral blood-vessels. In consequence there are relatively more old men who are mentally disturbed as the effect of a stroke, but their longer-lived wives are still there to look after them. Women, on the other hand, live on to develop the mental illnesses of extreme old age and have often outlived their husbands and other relatives, so hospital admission is frequently required.

*Roth, M. and Kay, D. W. K. (1962) Social, medical and personal factors associated with vulnerability to psychiatric breakdown in old age. *Geront. clin.* 4, 147–160.

The Influence of Physical Illness

There is a close connection between physical and mental illness in old people. Mental illness may sometimes be the direct result of a physical condition (as in the example given above of the after-effects of a stroke) or it may appear in association with physical illness, especially if the latter is chronic, debilitating or painful. Sensory defects such as blindness or deafness are important as they may cut the elderly person off from contact with other people and from sources of information and amusement such as newspapers, radio and television. Reduced mobility due to stiffening joints and increasing weakness have the same effect. Not uncommonly, psychiatric illness appears after the elderly person has had an operation: sometimes this takes the form of confusion due to the after-effects of the anaesthetic and the overwhelming effect of strange surroundings, but on other occasions it is a depressive illness which is precipitated by the operative procedure.

Effects of Environment

As a rule, isolation is bad for the old person. It probably depends on the individual as to whether he does better with young company or with people of his own generation, but he does need other human company. If he is vigorous and maintains his interests he can get out regularly to meet others, but if he is at all restricted, companionship and care must be brought to him. Sometimes the husband or wife is able to provide all that is required, but as elderly couples become feebler they may need regular supervision. The possibility of accidents and gassing have to be remembered, and during winter the danger of hypothermia due to inadequate heating is a very real one. Diet is very important and some aged people become mentally ill as the result of malnutrition and consequent severe vitamin deficiency.

Bereavement of a close relative may have severe effects on an old person. Often there is no profound grief when a husband or wife dies because the emotions become greatly diminished with advanced age, but the survivor may find it impossible to change long-established habits and may pine away when left alone. The accustomed patterns of family life (including eating habits) are no longer there to sustain and comfort.

Effect of the Previous Personality

In the study by Roth and Kay which we have already mentioned some of the findings suggested that old people who were socially isolated and mentally disturbed had not infrequently had odd personalities throughout their adult lives and this had been an important factor in making them solitary. So, in some cases, loneliness may be an expression of mental abnormality rather than a cause. As well as this, the person who has had an abnormally rigid personality before reaching old age will have greater than average difficulty in adjusting to the changes in existence brought about by retirement and increasing feebleness.

At times the person may have been seriously mentally disturbed long before old age, but senility exaggerates the condition. Often this type of person comes to notice only when the relative who has been caring for him dies and leaves him totally unable to fend for himself.

Neurotic Illnesses of Old Age

It is now time to consider the individual conditions. Since there is evidence that psychoneurosis is probably one of the commonest maladies of the elderly it would seem logical to begin with a detailed discussion of it: unfortunately information is extremely scanty. We know that neurosis in the elderly can take several forms. Elderly people may suffer from various forms of reactive or neurotic depression which are often quite chronic and these may cause the sufferer to be complaining and cantankerous. Anxiety is a very common symptom and at times may take the form of panic attacks. Phobic symptoms are not uncommon and they often have a fairly realistic basis: the old person may be afraid to go downstairs lest he fall or may be afraid of noises in the dark in case they might be caused by burglars. It is often difficult to be sure about obsessional symptoms in the psychiatric sense since at this age people are normally fairly obsessional, but preoccupation with ill-health is very common. The old person is often fanatically interested in the state of his bowels and self-medication is very common. Sometimes this amounts to a state of severe hypochondriasis with multiple physical complaints. Many old people are disturbed atbout the imminence of death: some appear to take a morbid pleasure in its occurrence in others and one occasionally comes across the elderly individual who almost gleefully ticks off each of his contemporaries as they predecease him! This feeling of personal invincibility probably prevents too much introspection about his own impending death.

The old person often needs less sleep than he did when he was young but complaints of insomnia are very common. Night-time is frequently a time of restlessness and anxiety, sometimes of confusion. Sleeping-drugs are often required, but care must be taken in their use: they may increase the patient's confusion and, in some old people, they may tend to cause restlessness rather than rest.

The possibility of these neurotic illnesses being present should always be considered. It is too easy to attribute everything to the inescapable effects of old age when, in some cases at least, the old person may be suffering unnecessarily. In many instances the neurotic symptoms represent a break-down in the old person's defences against difficult circumstances and treatment will consist more of practical help and supervision than of psychotherapy and drugs. Ensuring that the old person is physically as well as possible also removes the root cause of many neurotic symptoms. Treatment should be directed towards helping the patient to live more happily and more self-sufficiently.

Psychotic Conditions in Old Age

We have a good deal more information about the psychotic illnesses since so many of these patients require admission to hospital. Nowadays it is considered highly important that old people with severe mental illness be thoroughly assessed because it is known that a considerable proportion are suffering from illnesses which will respond well to treatment.

Roth (1955)* examined the records of a hospital population of elderly psychotic patients and found that, with few exceptions, they fell into five main categories. These categories are (1) Affective disorder, (2) Senile dementia, (3) Arteriosclerotic dementia (due to hardening of the cerebral arteries), (4) Acute confusional states, (5) Late paraphrenia. In order to plan a social work approach it is necessary to know what is likely to happen to these old people after their admission to hospital.

When the different groups were followed up after two years their fate was found to be as follows:

1. Affective disorder   60 per cent discharged
2. Senile dementia   80 per cent dead
3. Arteriosclerotic dementia 70 per cent dead
4. Acute confusional states   50 per cent dead: 50 per cent discharged
5. Late paraphrenia   More than half still in hospital

So far as can be made out, the functional psychoses of old age and the psychoses caused by organic deterioration of the brain appear to be relatively independent of each other, though sometimes an illness will show features of both.

1. *Affective Disorder*

This is now realized to be one of the commonest psychiatric illnesses of old age and it usually takes the form of depression rather than of mania. There is often an admixture of symptoms of anxiety, agitation and hypochondriasis. The depression may be a recurrence of an illness which first appeared in earlier life but it not uncommonly arises for the first time after the age of 60. It may occur in various degrees of severity: if it is very severe and if the patient becomes very retarded he may appear to be demented. Suicide is not uncommon in this condition, especially in men.

Depression which appears for the first time in old age is often precipitated by an acute stress such as physical illness, bereavement,

---

*Roth, M. (1955) The natural history of mental disorder in old age. *J. ment. Sci.* **101**, 281.

injury or operation, but this stress commonly arises out of a chronic illness which has been present for a considerable time. Sensory deficits (blindness and deafness) are frequently in evidence in these cases and any treatment should include dealing with these. The mortality rate is higher in the late onset group because of the associated physical illness factors than it is in those whose illness is simply a recurrence of an earlier depression.

It always has to be remembered that in some cases of depression there is an underlying element of dementia. This may be seen in the patient who is depressed and who also has a raised blood-pressure and hardening of the cerebral arteries. In these cases the mood is usually not fixed at a depressed level but is extremely labile: at times the patient is extremely morose and at others he is facile and facetious. The suicide rate is high in such patients.

The response to antidepressant treatment is usually so good in an uncomplicated case and the difference in the patient's state of well-being is often so extraordinary that it is tragic to overlook the condition. Often it is necessary to treat the person in hospital, partly because of the risk of suicide in the acute stages and partly because of the possibility of side-effects from the treatment which tend to be more severe in the aged. During the stay in hospital the old person often frets and worries about what is happening to his or her home, to the pet cat and a hundred and one other little things. Good social work at this stage may markedly shorten the individual's period of agitation and depression. On return home it is hoped that the patient will become independent again but regular supportive visits are valuable, both to check progress and to provide company.

2. Late Paraphrenia

This is possibly a rather mixed group of patients, but a considerable proportion appear to be suffering from schizophrenia of late onset. In the elderly this usually assumes the paranoid form (see p. 225). Late paraphrenia is much commoner in the unmarried (especially unmarried women) and in the divorced, but is not especially frequent amongst the widowed. The people who suffer from it often appear to live to a great age and it has been suggested that in some cases it is mainly the patient's extreme longevity and consequent isolation from contemporaries who have predeceased him that have precipitated the illness.

Certainly it sometimes appears as though the illness has been brought on by the death of a relative or by a disability such as deafness aggravating loneliness, but, on the other hand, many patients with late paraphrenia have suffered from chronic forms of personality disorder, especially of the schizoid type, long before they became old. It is likely that the abnormal personality has been the cause of the celibacy and the loneliness which are so often found in association with the illness.

The patients usually complain that they are being persecuted in some persistent manner and not infrequently there are bizarre sexual overtones to their complaints. Hallucinations are common and the patient may claim that the neighbours are being deliberately noisy or people are forever flashing lights through the window at night or someone is planting dead rats under the floorboards to cause an unpleasant smell. Sometimes he may cause a considerable disturbance by shouting back at the imaginary voices or repeatedly telephoning the police to report various outrages. Sometimes the complaints are taken seriously at first because in other ways the person is often mentally well preserved, alert and well orientated.

Treatment may depend on the amount of co-operation one can get from the patient, and the necessity for treatment depends more on the degree of social disturbance that she is causing than on the actual severity of the illness: a very deluded old lady who keeps her strange beliefs to herself may be able to remain in the community whereas a much less disturbed individual who makes a great fuss about her imaginary persecutions may have to be admitted to hospital. If the person can stay at home every attempt should be made to deal with defects such as deafness, and if she has to be on drugs she must be persuaded to take them regularly. Home visiting such a patient may be a thankless task: it often consists of patiently listening to a tirade of complaints, occasionally slipping in a bland question and offering advice and help whenever it is possible.

If the patient has to enter hospital there is a considerable chance that her symptoms will fail to improve with treatment and many of these people have to remain inpatients for the rest of their lives. However, with one of the powerful tranquillizing drugs a proportion will respond sufficiently to be fit for discharge. Then a decision has to be made in each case whether it is wise to allow the patient to return to a relatively solitary existence or whether other suitable arrangements should be made for her, such as arranging admission to an old folk's home. Either way, a good deal of follow-up care will be required.

3. *Organic Psychoses in the Elderly: Delirium*

Elderly people are particularly liable to develop acute delirious illnesses in the course of other conditions: for example, as the result of organic damage to the brain or during an attack of more generalized physical disease. Often the story is that they have been enjoying good health and then they have suffered a condition such as heart failure, a mild cerebral thrombosis or pneumonia: thereafter they are precipitated into a confused mental state. Nowadays, another important cause of delirium is the prolonged taking of sleeping tablets, especially barbiturates: the old person's metabolism is much less efficient at dealing with these and they tend to accumulate gradually within the body. After a time they produce symptoms of confusion and not infrequently of restlessness. If restlessness and sleeplessness are prominent there is a danger that their cause will be overlooked and further drugs given in an attempt to counteract them. Quite commonly, as we have mentioned, confusion develops when the old person is taken into hospital, partly because of the after-effects of operation and partly because of unfamiliar surroundings.

The outstanding features of delirious illnesses are confusion, disorientation and memory disturbance, which may vary greatly in their severity from moment to moment. During the relatively confusion-free periods the patient often appears alert and well, but this should not engender a false sense of confidence since shortly afterwards he can become excited and deluded and may then wander away and come to some accidental grief.

The treatment of the mental state is the treatment of the underlying illness and the outlook for the patient depends on the nature of that illness. Medical and nursing care are required and nowadays with treatment a good number of these old people make a good recovery. When they are well again they may be fit to go home, but they will probably require the help of a number of social services: district nursing, meals on wheels, home visiting and so on. If the old person is kept alert, well fed and physically healthy he may enjoy a considerable period of useful life following recovery.

4. *Organic Psychoses in the Elderly: Dementia*

The outlook in the dementing illnesses is much less hopeful. Here, the brain is damaged or has deteriorated and in many instances the disorder is inexorably progressive. A high proportion of the patients die within a year or two and those who survive longer are often mere shells of their former selves. In effect the brain of a demented person has aged at a much greater rate than his body: until quite recently the usual outcome would have been a very rapid death due to inanition or an illness like pneumonia, but nowadays antibiotics and other treatments can keep at least the body alive. Doctors are often ethically unwilling to withhold such treatments although they know that in many cases the mental functions are destroyed for ever. Geriatric wards are accumulating ever-increasing numbers of elderly patients in this condition.

The two commonest dementias in the aged are the senile and arteriosclerotic types. In other cases dementia is often due to the results of systemic illness, cancer, etc.

Senile dementia. The brains of all old people tend to atrophy because of progressive loss of nerve cells, but this is normally such a gradual process that the individual usually compensates and death occurs before the mental effects are disastrous. In senile dementia the process of brain deterioration has gone rather more rapidly and for some reason (perhaps a strong physical constitution) the person has not died. This illness mostly occurs in people in their late sixties and beyond, and the symptoms usually progress gradually but unremittingly.

The mental activities become slower and memory (particularly for recent events) becomes more and more inadequate. The person is easily confused and this may cause outbursts of agitation, panic or anger. The social behaviour deteriorates and dress and appearance are neglected. Sometimes antisocial habits appear which are quite out of keeping with the previous personality: the old person may become gluttonous, or create disturbances or attempt to interfere sexually with children. Confusion may lead to episodes of wandering, especially at night. Sleep is often very disturbed although the individual may nod off at unlikely times during the day. Emotion becomes unstable, with alternating periods of euphoria with foolish behaviour and periods of depression and agitation. Delusions may develop and as a result of these the person may become very truculent and difficult to deal with. The patient often has no insight whatsoever into his disturbed state. Every so often he may develop an acute attack of delirium when all his symptoms worsen.

In a high proportion of cases the patient reaches a stage where he can no longer remain at home. Relatives should be encouraged and helped to keep him as long as possible, but often they are unwilling to tend a confused, restless, truculent old person who may well be incontinent and who may be a source of danger since he may totter around turning on gas taps, lighting matches and spilling boiling water. Where the relatives do agree to keep him at home they will often need a great deal of practical help and moral support.

Arteriosclerotic dementia. In this illness the psychological changes are due to brain damage brought about by disease of the cerebral blood vessels, often associated with high blood-pressure. Sometimes the deterioration is a fairly gradual process but in many cases there are intermittent episodes of brain damage due to a cerebral thrombosis or haemorrhage. A severe stroke will often cause death, but recovery from a less severe one, or a series of minor strokes is quite common nowadays. Consequently this form of dementia frequently comes on in a series of separate steps, with further mental deterioration following each stroke. The first signs of the illness may appear before old age in some individuals and then progress slowly. Due to the neurological damage which occurs there are often accompanying physical disabilities such as paralyses or epileptic attacks: the patient frequently complains of severe headache and buzzing in his ears and these may make him thoroughly miserable. At times there may be periods of acute confusion and delirium, usually when another episode involving brain damage has occurred.

The usual features of dementia appear: recent memory is usually impaired, there is slowing of intellectual function and social habits deteriorate. The emotions fluctuate a great deal and the person will readily become over-excited or irritable and periods of deep gloom and depression are common. He may become very difficult to live with, partly because he often retains some degree of insight into his numerous disabilities: he can appreciate how much his illness restricts him and this makes him extremely impatient with himself and with others. This insight also encourages depression and suicide is relatively common during fits of despair.

When the illness is severe the patient usually dies quite soon, but deterioration and death are not inevitable. Some cases have a good outcome, particularly when the underlying disease (for example, hypertension) can be treated and the brain damage has not progressed too far. In these cases, intensive treatment including drugs, physiotherapy for paralyses, and speech therapy may produce excellent results. Sometimes there is a remarkable amount of recovery of intellectual function and of the personality: antidepressant treatment is often of help here. However, even after a good recovery there may be some degree of physical or mental impairment and the person may require help to find suitable work and perhaps to adjust to a lower level of achievement. When the illness is progressive and the outlook poor, the relatives will require psychological and practical support, both when the patient is at home and during his terminal period in hospital.

5. *Suicide in the Elderly*

Although we deal with suicide in more detail elsewhere (see

Chapter 8) it is as well to emphasize that it occurs more commonly in the middle-aged and elderly than in any other age group.

Suicide in the aged appears to be associated with a number of factors: in particular, with social isolation, bereavement and the effects of retirement such as lack of useful employment and the loss of community status which work affords. It is also frequently associated with depression, the early stages of dementing illnesses, with disabling and debilitating physical disease and with deafness or blindness. Where the danger of suicide is realized, temporary hospitalization may forestall the act. If the old person is able to return home, the various social and medical factors we have mentioned will obviously need to be dealt with.

B. PSYCHOTIC ILLNESSES DUE TO ORGANIC CAUSES

We have been discussing mental illnesses of old age and we have pointed out that by no means all of them are due to organic deterioration of the brain. On the other hand, it is true to say that dementias and delirious conditions are most often associated nowadays with old age and its various attendant complications: yet organic psychiatric illnesses can and do occur at any age. We shall now describe the more important manifestations of the organic psychoses which appear before old age. As with senile organic states, they can be classified as delirium or dementia according to the possibility or not of recovery.

Delirium

This is an acute confusional state which is usually reversible unless the underlying disease cannot be halted. Delirium may be associated with disease or trauma to the brain itself, but in the majority of cases it is a complication of a more generalized acute physical illness. It has become much less common since antibiotic treatment has been introduced in severe infective conditions and since the importance of correcting biochemical abnormalities in acute illnesses has been realized. Delirious conditions are usually found in feverish illnesses and in illnesses where biochemical disturbance is prominent or where there is an accumulation of toxic substances in the blood-stream. They are also a feature of epilepsy in some individuals.

The most characteristic feature of delirium is a temporary change in the patient's state of consciousness: he enters a confused, dreamy state and is often disorientated to some extent as to time and place. Restlessness is frequent and sometimes there are outbursts of wild excitement or panic. On the other hand, retardation of thought and behaviour may be present, even to the extent of the patient becoming stuporose. The individual shows a good deal of bewilderment and may be quite markedly deluded. At times there may be hallucinations, often auditory or visual in nature. The symptoms commonly fluctuate considerably so that at times the patient appears quite calm and rational, then soon after becomes confused and disturbed again.

In very mild cases of confusion the condition may not be noticed. This can happen after a blow on the head which has caused some degree of concussion but no unconsciousness, or it may occur in a person who is suffering from the after-effects of an anaesthetic, perhaps after a visit to the dentist. Superficially the person appears normal, but if he is allowed to go off unsupervised he may do something irrational such as crossing a busy road with complete disregard of the traffic or wandering about in an aimless fashion. If he comes to no harm he often has little or no recollection of this episode.

The symptoms of delirium are usually acute enough to warrant medical supervision and treatment and in any case the patient is often in hospital on account of the underlying disorder. Today the illnesses which are most often associated with delirium include infections such as pneumonia and typhoid, and non-infectious disorders such as chronic kidney disease, jaundice due to severe liver disease, and a serious degree of heart failure. Acute disease of the brain such as encephalitis may produce similar mental symptoms and so may head injury, as we have already mentioned. On occasion there may be an episode of confusion preceding or following an epileptic seizure, but this is described in more detail below (see p.257).

At the present time, drugs (whether medically prescribed or otherwise) are a fairly common cause of confusional states. Barbiturates are consumed in enormous quantities in the general population: taken in excessive amounts or over a prolonged period they can cause chronic confusion not unlike a mild state of drunkenness. Various groups of people (for example, the youngster who wants to be "pepped up" or the chronically tired middle-aged housewife) take stimulants like amphetamine or dexamphetamine to provide extra energy: the effects are usually short-lived and there is a tendency to keep increasing the dose until, in some cases, an acute delirium is precipitated. Other drugs such as marijuana, mescaline or cocaine can also cause delirium in some individuals. Alcohol is well known for its immediate symptoms and these are often typical of an acute confusional state: in chronic alcoholics, delirium tremens (see p. 166) is a common complication of alcoholic abuse.

Delirium usually responds to treatment of the causative illness and, in itself, the condition does not require much intervention by the social worker. However, in those cases where the basic illness is not recoverable or where there are complications like alcoholism or drug addiction the social worker may become much involved in the treatment of the patient and his family.

Dementias

It is distressing to see an elderly person suffering from progressive mental illness due to brain deterioration, but at least it is consoling to know that he has lived his full life-span. It is much more tragic to witness a younger individual who suffers from irreversible brain damage: tragic as much from his family's point of view as from his own.

Dementia is a condition of psychological disturbance due to brain damage. The disturbance is to a great extent irreversible and may be progressive. Dementia may develop suddenly (as in some cases of head injury or encephalitis) or its appearance may be more gradual (as in cases due to arteriosclerosis or hardening of the cerebral arteries or as a late result of severe epilepsy in some individuals).

The main features of dementia have already been described in the section on the illness of old age (see p. 246). It is characterized by memory loss, often beginning with difficulty in remembering names, then progressing to severe forgetfulness, particularly with regard to recent events: in the later stages the patient is unable to retain fresh memories and also has great difficulty in recollecting events from the fairly recent past, but memory of the distant past is usually relatively unaffected till very late on. Thinking becomes slow and progressively more restricted in its range: abstract thought is severely impoverished and the individual's thinking gets into more and more of a rut. The emotions become unstable and fluctuate rapidly from euphoria to depression and from apathy to agitation. Sometimes there are periods of sustained elation or depression. Judgement is usually severely affected and social behaviour deteriorates: the person may become slovenly and careless of hygiene, gross and uninhibited in behaviour and he may commit various antisocial acts.

Delusions are common and take various forms. The patient may complain of persecution, accuse his wife of infidelity or develop grandiose notions. Hallucinations sometimes appear, especially when, as often happens, acute delirious episodes occur. The individual may be very restless and distractible, but often he is apathetic and loses all his drive and initiative. He easily becomes muddled, cannot make decisions and his work performance is drastically affected. Eventually he becomes disorientated and loses track of time and place.

If the dementia is due to some general physical disease there may be associated physical handicaps—for example, a paralysis due to a stroke or cirrhosis of the liver in chronic alcoholism. When the dementia reaches an advanced stage the patient often becomes physically debilitated and resistance to infection is greatly reduced. Incontinence may develop and it is often at this stage that the relatives find it impossible to cope. Epilepsy sometimes appears as a result of the brain damage and it too gives rise to very considerable social difficulties.

Naturally any patient who is suspected of becoming demented

must be thoroughly examined both physically and psychologically. There are various psychological tests which can demonstrate deterioration in intellect and aptitudes and these are of great value in detecting the early and still doubtful case. The more advanced cases present with such obvious symptoms that the diagnosis of dementia is readily made, but every case is assessed physically to discover whether a potentially treatable condition is present, such as excessively high blood-pressure, a removable brain tumour or an infection of the brain like syphilis. Whenever dementia is suspected every effort should be made to establish an early diagnosis: if treatment is possible it would be regrettable to allow brain damage to continue. Once the dementing process has begun some permanent damage will have occurred, but after treatment there is often a considerable recovery of function. However, even in successful cases recuperation is usually slow, there may well be residual disabilities and the patient may require a great deal of social help during his rehabilitation process.

Unfortunately many of the dementing conditions are not susceptible to medical treatment and the deterioration progresses, sometimes slowly but sometimes very quickly. For example, the dementia which at times accompanies multiple sclerosis may develop gradually over a period of ten years, whereas in some cases of hypertension the dementia runs a rapid course and the patient may die within a few months. Sometimes the dementia is severe, but non-progressive, as may occur after a serious head injury. In any case, relatives are going to need a great deal of help to accept the extremely distressing situation: it is often very difficult to explain to the patient's family that he is never going to recover his faculties and the difficulty is made much greater when, as sometimes happens, he appears physically well. Once the family has accepted the situation medical and social help should be provided to enable the patient to remain at home for as long as possible. In most cases admission to hospital is ultimately necessary and when this occurs there is scope for valuable supportive social work to aid the relatives and for liaison work between the family and the hospital.

Some Specific Organic Cerebral Conditions

The person who is suffering from the effects of a chronic dementing illness presents many social problems. He is unlikely to be able to carry on at his usual work and may well be unable to continue as the family breadwinner. His behaviour may be unpredictable and difficult and his treatment may involve his family in much time and trouble. By discussing briefly a few of the commoner of these conditions we hope to illustrate some of these difficulties.

  1. *The after-effects of head injury.* Immediately after a mild head injury there may be no more than headache and perhaps momentary dazing. A rather more severe head injury may produce concussion in which marked confusion can occur: at times this may not be detected and it is only afterwards when the individual has recovered and he realizes that he has had a period of amnesia that it becomes obvious that his consciousness was affected. An even more serious head injury is likely to cause unconsciousness, and on recovery from this there is often a period of delirium with considerable confusion which may last for a variable time. There is often amnesia for much of the post-injury confusional period and there may also be amnesia for the time immediately preceding the accident. As well as this, if the brain has been severely damaged it is likely that there will be a number of neurological effects, possibly including paralysis, speech disturbances, etc. In these cases neurosurgical treatment is often necessary.

The severer type of head injury is frequently associated with psychological damage. Nowadays this has become an important problem: brain damage can occur as a result of car accidents, industrial accidents, sporting accidents and so on. Surgeons can now save the lives of patients who would formerly have died as a result of such injuries. Unconscious patients can be kept alive for many months until consciousness returns, but unfortunately there is no guarantee that the severely brain-damaged individual will always make an adequate psychological recovery.

Even where intellectual deterioration is not obvious the person who survives a serious head injury may show some degree of personality change. There is often a reduction in emotional drive and in general efficiency. The individual may be more distractible and irritable than previously and his mood may become quite labile. In some cases depression is severe and may develop into a true depressive illness: in others a schizophrenic illness may appear. It is thought that in these cases a constitutional predisposition was present and was evoked by the effects of the injury. Often there are persistent complaints of headache and giddiness and some patients become extremely hypochondriacal. Irritability in some cases may erupt into attacks of aggression, even to the extent of violence, and in some individuals this may be associated with irresponsibility and lack of remorse to such a degree that the personality could almost be labelled "psychopathic".

All the symptoms of post-traumatic personality change may become inextricably mixed with the symptoms of the so-called compensation neurosis. Many of these individuals are involved in civil litigation to obtain damages for their injuries and consciously or unconsciously they frequently prolong and exaggerate their symptoms in order to obtain the maximum recompense. Sometimes this is plain malingering but usually the person is relatively unaware of his motives: nevertheless he clings to his symptoms till they become habitual and by the time the case is settled more damage may have been done to the personality than was originally caused by the injury.

In addition to personality changes there may sometimes be actual intellectual damage as a result of head injury. The person's intelligence level falls and this is often associated with defects of memory, poor concentration, difficulty in abstract thinking and a reduced capacity for problem-solving. Not uncommonly some insight is retained, but this is often just enough to make the individual unhappy and not enough to enable him to adapt to his new limitations. At times he clings stubbornly to his former aspirations though it is obvious to everyone else that he cannot possibly succeed: he himself denies his difficulties, but becomes more and more morose as he repeatedly fails. Suicide is not uncommon in this situation.

The person's difficulties may be compounded by the development of epilepsy. This occurs most commonly where there has been a penetrating injury to the brain or where a portion of the skull has been pushed inwards by a blow and has damaged the underlying brain substance. Sometimes the personality changes resulting from injury make it difficult for the patient to co-operate in anti-convulsant treatment and this may make control of the fits very difficult.

After a severe head injury the person needs a period of recuper-ation and rehabilitation which involves physical, psychological and social factors and which must be co-ordinated to promote the maximum degree of recovery. Part of the rehabilitation process consists of helping the patient to adapt to his various disabilities and helping the family to cope with someone whose personality and capabilities are so changed that, in some instances, he is virtually a different person. Both patient and family will need skilled help in enabling him to adapt to a new occupation and to a new way of life. The problem is long-term, but in many cases the patient gradually recovers function over a period of several years and careful handling will help him to realize his new maximum poten-tial. Quite often psychiatric treatment is required: at times psycho-therapy to help the patient with his emotional problems, at other times antidepressant treatment or tranquillizers. With an active approach there are relatively few head-injury victims who cannot be expected to respond in some way.

2. *Epilepsy.* We want to stress that the great majority of epileptics are people who are perfectly normal apart from their fits. Nowadays in most cases the fits can be well controlled to the point where, with drugs, they may entirely cease. Nevertheless the epileptic does have an unusually difficult life in many ways: his choice of occupation is restricted by the need to avoid heights or dangerous machinery, he should not drive a car, and his illness may so frighten people that he is turned into something of an outcast. Understand-ably some epileptics develop neurotic reactions to their problems and may require support or treatment on this account. Special societies and social clubs for the epileptic often have a marked

morale-boosting effect because in this situation he can feel that he is one of a group.

Epilepsy can occur for the first time at any age. It may appear spontaneously or may be due to numerous causes such as head injury, brain infection or tumour: in the great majority of cases the cause is benign and non-progressive. Not all epilepsy takes the form of generalized convulsions (known as Grand Mal epilepsy). Some forms occur as localized convulsions, perhaps of an arm or a leg, and some, known as Petit Mal, consist not of convulsions at all, but of brief periods of mental blankness (called Absences) during which the patient usually does not respond to stimuli. Epilepsy arises as the result of abnormal functioning of a portion of the brain and the form the epilepsy takes depends largely on the situation of that abnormal portion.

Change of consciousness is a usual but not invariable feature of the attacks in the various types of epilepsy. Sometimes consciousness is altered before or after as well as during the attack. Before the seizure occurs many patients experience a premonitory sensation known as the Aura. This may be a headache, an abdominal sensation, a feeling of impending doom or sometimes an irrational act of which the person has no recollection afterwards. After a generalized seizure there is often a period of confusion during which the patient may wander. In some cases there is no actual fit and its place is taken by an episode of dream-like confusion and disturbed behaviour very similar to a delirious illness but usually shorter-lived.

Possibly about half of all epileptics have seizures which originate in the region of the brain immediately underlying the temple-bone. This type of disorder is known as temporal lobe epilepsy and is frequently associated with both short-term and long-term psychological disturbances. Some individuals show very marked mood-swings and may on occasion be irritable or violent. Chronic hypochondriasis is quite common and sometimes persecutory delusions occur. These symptoms may be intermingled with disturbances of memory or of learning ability. At times there may be generalized convulsions or much more limited seizures associated with altered consciousness and a state which, in some ways, resembles sleep-walking.

In all cases of epilepsy the medical practitioner should attempt to find the cause or at least demonstrate that the illness is not due to some progressive lesion. In most cases the treatment is symptomatic and is designed to stop the seizures without necessarily removing the cause: various anticonvulsant drugs are used for this purpose with great success. Sometimes epilepsy is due to a condition in which surgical treatment is more appropriate and in this instance the surgeon will attempt to remove the abnormal portion of brain. If the operation is completely successful the epilepsy will cease and the patient will be able to lead a normal life. However, in some cases the surgeon may unavoidably cause a certain amount of damage to surrounding brain tissue in removing the lesion: then the patient may develop neurological defects which are usually minor but will necessitate a period of skilled rehabilitation.

In a small proportion of epileptics there is progressive brain damage, either because the seizures themselves are unduly severe or because the patient suffers repeated head injuries due to falls during fits. (Recently it has come to be realized that some anticonvulsant drugs can interfere with the absorption of certain vitamins and, if given over a long period, can also lead to the development of mental symptoms or even dementia.) The brain-damaged epileptic often displays a slowly advancing deterioration of intellect and memory and in a few cases this can proceed to a state of severe dementia. As well as this he may undergo marked changes of personality. Typically his thinking becomes sluggish and circumstantial, while conversation is garrulous and repetitive. The patient is often superficially ingratiating, but underneath he is stubborn, awkward and provocative. Self-righteousness, pomposity and religiosity are common and suspiciousness amounting to paranoia may be found. If this last feature is marked it may lead to the individual's admission to a psychiatric hospital and most mental hospitals contain a group of such "Epileptic Personalities". However, it is important to note that, as regards epilepsy as a whole, such severe abnormalities are uncommon and they should become even less frequent as modern treatment prevents brain damage in more and more epileptics. It is worth making this point because psychiatric text-books often give the impression that psychological deterioration is common in epilepsy and this is no longer necessarily true.

However, it cannot be denied that some epileptics are particularly difficult people who go through life with many imaginary grudges in addition to their undoubtedly real ones. These individuals are often unco-operative and unreliable in taking their medicines and they require a great deal of supervision and support in their work, in their family life and in their relations with other people. Supervision is often a thankless task, but every attempt should be made to prevent these people from becoming chronic institutional inmates. To ensure this there must be close co-operation between general practitioner, neurologist, psychiatrist and social worker.

3. *Pre-senile dementias.* These are a group of illnesses in which typical signs of dementia occur before old age. They arise from a variety of causes: some rare conditions are hereditary (for example, Alzheimer's disease and Niemann–Pick's disease) and these usually get a large section devoted to them in text-books because they provide many points of interest to doctors. However, as well as being uncommon they are untreatable and the patient usually deteriorates fairly rapidly. More common causes of pre-senile dementia include infections of the brain such as syphilis and encephalitis; generalized diseases like multiple sclerosis, hypertension and chronic under-activity of the thyroid gland (myxoedema); and damage to the brain caused by tumours or by trauma. So far as the social worker is concerned the causal factors are to a great extent academic, and what matters in each case is whether the condition can be regarded as static or progressive, acute or chronic, treatable or untreatable, since the part played by social work will depend on such factors.

In the rapidly progressive types of dementia the patient quickly becomes incapable of looking after himself and he needs mostly medical and nursing care: in these circumstances it is the family which requires intensive social supervision, usually in the form of financial and practical help for the spouse and the children. In the more chronic forms of the illness the patient's employers may have to be asked for their co-operation to enable the individual to remain at work as long as possible, even though he will have to undertake less onerous and less productive types of task. If the patient has associated physical disabilities, difficulties regarding accommodation and travel may arise. The patient may have a slight degree of insight and often this makes him irritable, depressed and difficult to live with. If this occurs psychiatric help may be required. However, the social worker's most important and most demanding task lies in providing the sort of psychological support to the patient's family which will enable them to adapt to the distressing spectacle of a close relative rapidly going downhill and dying at a comparatively early age.

CHAPTER 11

Psychiatry, the Law and the Community

THROUGHOUT this book we have stressed that mind and body are not separate entities but are aspects of the total person which are mutually interactive and interdependent. Illness of the body affects the workings of the mind and illness of the mind produces repercussions on the body and some of these repercussions are measureable. For example, when an individual is particularly anxious it is well known that his pulse-rate and blood-pressure rise. The mind is a highly complex function of brain activity and its complexity makes it seem mysterious, but nowadays its mysteries are yielding little by little to research. As this happens, it becomes obvious that psychiatric illness is no more extraordinary or morally reprehensible than physical illness. The general public is coming to accept this change of belief. The fact that something can undoubtedly be done to help many psychiatric patients has engendered a feeling of optimism and this in turn has made it respectable to suffer from psychiatric illness, or at least to admit to the world that one is suffering in this way. A patient no longer enters a psychiatric hospital because he has become insane. Instead, he is much more likely to seek medical advice in the earlier and milder stages of a nervous disorder. We must not give the false impression that psychiatry is all-healing or is able to create new personalities, and we hope that we have already doused this over-optimistic view. Nevertheless it is undoubtedly true that psychiatry has made extremely important advances in recent years and methods are becoming steadily more effective. This being so, it is especially important that the social worker should keep abreast of the rapid progress of knowledge and therapeutic efficiency.

The Mental Health Acts

Until the passing of the Mental Health Act, 1959 (in Scotland, the Mental Health (Scotland) Act, 1960), the law assumed that the majority of psychiatric patients would need inpatient care. Until a few years before these Acts were passed a very high proportion of patients were admitted under certification to mental hospital because their illness had reached a stage at which disturbed behaviour was occurring. After the Second World War this situation radically altered and there was growing emphasis on outpatient treatment and on psychiatric treatment in general hospitals. Because of this, more stress was laid on the necessity for the early recognition and treatment of mental illness. With the increase in the variety and effectiveness of treatment it became much more possible to treat patients outside the mental hospital and even to carry therapy into the community itself. The Mental Health Acts were passed in recognition of these important trends. They repealed all the foregoing legislation on mental illness and mental subnormality and they declared that treatment should always be on a voluntary basis unless circumstances made this impossible. The Acts also made treatment in most cases "informal", so that the individual undergoing psychiatric treatment is no more under legal restraint than the one receiving treatment for a physical disorder. Restriction of a patient's liberty is only permissible when his state of mind is so disturbed that he is a danger to himself or to the community, and even then the psychiatrist's power to insist on hospitalization and treatment is subject to proper limitations. The Mental Health Acts lay down that there should be an increasing amount of treatment at community level and they give local authorities a considerable responsibility for instituting various services which should have a close liaison with the psychiatric service and the general practitioner in the care and treatment of the psychiatrically ill. For example, the local authority is expected to provide residential accommodation for the patient who has just been discharged from hospital and who is not yet ready to enter a full life in the general community, for elderly people who are mentally infirm but not ill enough to require hospital treatment, and for educationally subnormal and maladjusted children who need care and supervision. It has a statutory responsibility nowadays to set up occupational and training centres for children who are unfit for an ordinary school education and for adults who are unable to work even in sheltered employment. The Acts also stress the desirability of the local authority's instituting ancillary and welfare services, day centres, social clubs and home visiting services.

Unfortunately, lack of funds and sometimes lack of interest or energy have resulted in some local authorities being less than enthusiastic in providing many of the services that the Acts visualized. Sometimes there has been a notable lack of co-operation with the psychiatric hospitals, often as much due to the fault of the hospital as of the authority. This has the unfortunate effect that many patients leave hospital and do not receive an adequate amount of social rehabilitation so that they break down once more and may have to re-enter hospital. As we shall mention shortly, there is an enormous field for co-operation between psychiatric and community services which is only just beginning to be tackled.

Another section of the Acts provides that Mental Welfare Officers (in Scotland, Mental Health Officers) will be appointed by the local authorities to undertake certain responsibilities in respect of psychiatric patients. The Mental Welfare Officer is involved in the procedure for admitting patients compulsorily to hospital who are in a disturbed state and he has certain statutory duties which include the authority to convey patients to hospital if they require compulsory admission, to return to the hospital patients who have been admitted on order and who have absconded, and to inspect premises where it is suspected that a mentally ill individual is present and is not receiving proper care. He may also be concerned with the aftercare of patients discharged from hospital, particularly where the local authority is responsible for, or has an interest in, the patient. In practice he is often so fully taken up with the strictly statutory aspects of his work that he has relatively little time for adequate follow-up care. As well as this, he is frequently involved with the more difficult type of patient whose illness has demanded compulsory admission to hospital, whose prognosis may not be very good and whose degree of co-operativeness following discharge is limited. These cases demand a great deal of individual care if repeated re-admission to hospital is to be avoided, but the busy Mental Welfare Officer is often too over-stretched to be able to provide this type of supervision. This is a great pity since he often has much useful experience and also valuable working arrangements with other branches of the local authority. These assets could well be shared with psychiatric and social work colleagues, and when the Mental Welfare Officer is included as a member of the therapeutic team he has a definite part to play in the rehabilitation of the patient and in dealing with the practical details of resettling him in the community.

Legal Definitions of Mental Illness

The proportion of patients who nowadays require admission under compulsory procedures is small. The vast majority of psychiatric disorders are not in any case associated with any form of disturbed behaviour which might necessitate the patient's restraint. In those illnesses which may eventually become florid it should often be possible to recognize the disorder at an early stage and intervene with treatment before the patient's insight and behaviour are excessively disordered. Even when an individual is unco-operative and is obviously mentally ill, every attempt is made to persuade him to accept treatment on an informal basis. If persuasion is unavailing and the patient is endangering himself or others, then there may be no alternative but to compel him to enter hospital. Danger to himself may take an active form if he threatens suicide, or may be passive if he is so incapacitated mentally that he cannot take adequate care of himself. Danger to others may arise if he becomes violent or if he creates some kind of public nuisance and cannot be dissuaded from doing this. When lack of insight prevents him from recognizing that he is ill and when he refuses treatment or consistently fails to co-operate, then it is obviously logical to treat him compulsorily.

The Mental Health Act, 1959, recognizes four categories of mental disorder for administrative purposes, and when compulsory admission is being carried out the psychiatrist must state the category of disorder from which the patient is suffering. The types of disorders are as follows:

Mental illness. This includes all forms of psychoneurotic and psychotic disorders. In practice, nearly all the patients who require admission against their own (irrational) wishes are suffering from illnesses such as schizophrenia, epileptic psychosis, very severe depression with a marked risk of suicide and dementias in which the individual has lost the ability to care for himself. It is rare for alcoholics or drug addicts to be compelled to enter hospital since their periods of acute irrationality are usually fairly circumscribed.

Psychopathic disorder. This is defined as a "Persistent disorder or disability of mind (whether or not including subnormality of intelligence) resulting in abnormally aggressive or seriously irresponsible conduct, requiring medical treatment".

Subnormality/severe subnormality. We are not concerned at present with these conditions. (N.B. The Scottish Act includes these two categories as one.)

It is worth noting that when a psychopath enters a psychiatric hospital he often does so for treatment of some additional psychiatric disability such as psychoneurosis and admission is usually informal. A relatively small proportion are admitted compulsorily because of the psychopathy itself. The Acts make special provisions for severely antisocial psychopaths to be detained in special institutions for the criminally insane or to receive psychiatric treatment in prison. (They also provide for the treatment of the non-psychopathic prisoner who is psychiatrically disturbed.)

Admission to a Psychiatric Hospital

As we have indicated, most patients today are admitted informally to hospital and this means that they maintain their full rights as citizens and that their legal position is almost exactly the same as that of the individual who enters hospital with a physical illness. In fact, in many instances the two types of patient will be admitted to adjoining wards in the same hospital. The informal psychiatric patient is entitled to leave hospital when he wishes, against medical advice if he insists. Occasionally it is evident that the patient is too disturbed to leave, and if this is so a senior member of the psychiatric staff can recommend detention for three days under Section 30 of the Acts. If the disturbed mental state clears up rapidly the compulsory order need not be extended, but if the patient remains very unwell the psychiatrist can initiate the procedure for keeping him in hospital for a further period. This procedure under Section 30 is rarely invoked and it is only an occasional patient who is so utterly insightless and dangerous (or helpless) whose liberty has to be curtailed in this way.

If compulsory admission is necessary, this is normally carried out only after the nearest relative has made application to the hospital for the patient to be admitted and after a medical practitioner has failed to persuade the patient to seek treatment. If the nearest relative is not available or if the case is so urgent that it is impracticable to go through the usual procedure, a Mental Welfare Officer can make the application, but except under unusual circumstances his application can be invalidated if the relative appears and refuses to sanction the admission. It is no longer necessary to seek a magistrate's permission to have the patient admitted on an order, but in normal circumstances two medical practitioners must recommend that admission is necessary and for this purpose they must have examined the patient within the 14 days prior to the date of the application. One of these practitioners should preferably be on the local authority's list of approved doctors with special experience in psychiatry and the other should be either the patient's general practitioner or the doctor who is looking after him in hospital.

There are three types of application for compulsory admission. The first, under Section 25 of the Acts, allows the hospital to detain the patient for 28 days for observational treatment. Many individuals recover sufficiently within this period to allow of their becoming informal patients, but if they still require compulsory treatment after four weeks the hospital must arrange for a further application to be made, this time under Section 26. This Section deals with all patients suffering from mental illness and severe subnormality and makes special provisions for psychopathic and subnormal individuals. These last two groups may be compulsorily admitted until the age of 21 on account of psychopathy or subnormality alone, but not thereafter, though if they are already in hospital and need to be detained there the order may be extended till they reach the age of 25. (After that, if they remain dangerous or unable to fend for themselves, special procedures have to be invoked.) The third type of application is under Section 29, and this allows three days of compulsory observation in the case of an emergency. The application in this case is made by the Mental Welfare Officer or any relative and need be accompanied by only one medical recommendation. If the patient still refuses to undergo treatment on an informal basis, the application may be converted to one under Section 25 by arranging for a second medical examination and recommendation to be made before the three-day period is up.

The law takes great care to ensure that the provisions of the Mental Health Acts are not abused and there is little or no substance to the layman's fear that he could be committed to a psychiatric hospital against his will when he is not suffering from a mental illness. Even when a patient is obviously deranged, Mental Welfare Officers and psychiatrists are still at pains to avoid compulsory procedures if at all possible. If the individual does have to be admitted to hospital on an order the law requires that the order be reviewed at regulated intervals. After a stated period he can protest to a Mental Health Tribunal, set up by the Act in order to protect the patient's interests. The nearest relative can, at any time, demand the patient's discharge at 72 hours' notice and this must be accepted unless an extremely good case can be made out against his leaving hospital.

Note

You will have noticed that we have given much more detail in our description of compulsory procedures than we have in discussing informal admission and treatment. The latter needs little explanation because it is so simple and straightforward. The former needs to be given detailed mention in order to reassure social workers who are not closely connected with the psychiatric field that there really has been a profound departure from former practice. The rights of the individual, even if he is suffering from a severe mental illness, are jealously guarded by the law and the law is adhered to by psychiatrists. The Mental Health Acts became possible when the outlook of psychiatry and of the public became more enlightened, but this enlightenment, as we have already said, could only come about because the effectiveness of treatment had reached a point at which it was possible to treat most psychiatric patients on the same basis as any other ill person.

Trends in the Psychiatric Services

The National Health Service provides a comprehensive system of care which ensures that anyone with a psychiatric disorder will receive treatment. On average it is probably as good a psychiatric service as one may find in most countries but it is by no means perfect. There is a gulf between the general practitioner and the hospital sections of the Health Service so that most general practitioners work in an atmosphere of professional isolation, cut off from hospital facilities and from contact with specialist colleagues. This often means that the general practitioner can only treat an illness to a certain point and then he has to pass the patient to the hospital where he can no longer take an active interest in his progress. This is a discouraging situation for a competent and interested doctor because so many of his cases disappear from his ken at a stage where he might obtain some satisfaction from seeing improvement occur. As well as this, the general practitioner is involved in many routine and repetitive tasks which rob him of the time and energy to carry out his proper function as a family practitioner. This is a great pity, particularly when it comes to psychiatric illness, since the family situation may be of considerable importance in certain aspects of such illness.

The great mass of psychiatric complaints is dealt with by the general practitioner, many of whom qualified before psychiatry could boast much in the way of active therapy. A good many of the older general practitioners admit that they are not in touch with modern advances in psychiatry, yet they still have to deal with the enormous numbers of depressed, anxious, insomniac or disturbed patients who present for treatment. Psychiatric education has greatly improved in recent years, but it still needs to reach many within the medical profession, general practitioners and non-psychiatric specialists alike, who remain only dimly aware of the frequency and disabling nature of psychiatric disorders and who do not appreciate the varying guises in which these disorders may appear. Many psychological disturbances are relatively minor and can be dealt with at a symptomatic level by reassurance or by simple drug therapy, or at a social level where some environmental difficulty can be alleviated. If the general practitioner had more knowledge and more time and if he had access to the appropriate facilities (including social work help and local authority services), a great many more patients could be treated very satisfactorily at home at a stage of their illness when no serious complications had arisen and with a minimum of disturbance to their way of life.

The psychiatrist used to be almost as confined to the mental hospital as his patients, but nowadays he may well work in a general hospital and have outpatient clinics in the community, sometimes in hospital and sometimes in conjunction with the local authority. Patients are being referred in ever-increasing numbers and there is nowadays a huge turn-over of outpatients and inpatients. Different facilities have been devised to suit various types of patient, including day hospitals, occupational centres and specialized units for alcoholics, drug addicts, psychopaths and others. There is a great need for other types of facility—for example, to deal with children and adolescents. It is much easier and much less anxiety-provoking for the patient than ever before to have psychiatric treatment, and psychiatric hospitals and clinics are far from being the fearsome places they once were. Despite this there are many psychiatrists who believe that the speciality is still too hospital-bound. There will always be a need for inpatient facilities in the foreseeable future for those who are extremely ill or disturbed (and for the growing numbers of elderly patients), but there is a very great need for community psychiatry. There must be closer links between the psychiatrist and the general practitioner and the sharing of facilities which, as we have said, would include the availability of social work help in general practice. There must also be a much closer liaison with the local authorities' mental health and allied services. The present arrangement means that there is a great deal of discontinuity in the handling of the patient. His illness has to be recognized, diagnosed and treated and then he may have to undergo rehabilitation and re-training. He may receive help from, among others, the general practitioner, the psychiatrist, the social worker, the Mental Welfare Officer, the district nurse, the Ministry of Labour and the Ministry of Social Security. All of this reflects a sophisticated standard of care, but between each stage of the process there is an ever-present danger that communication may break down to the detriment of the patient. Co-ordination of all these services is a necessity which, we hope, will not be neglected much longer.

As regards the social worker's position in relation to psychiatry, we would repeat what we have already said. The progressive psychiatrist values the social worker as a colleague who has special skills and who plays an important part in the assessment and re-habilitation of the patient, who sometimes participates actively in the treatment situation, and who is expert in dealing with and advising on the environmental aspects of the case. Admittedly some psychiatrists do not yet appreciate the function of the social worker, but we believe that their number is rapidly dwindling.

Psychiatry has changed radically in the past few years and on the whole it has changed greatly for the better. The rapid development in our methods has meant that psychiatrists themselves have had to reappraise their attitudes and have had to discard many obsolete concepts and methods. Those of us in academic psychiatry are concerned that the significance of these changes be made apparent to all medical practitioners, and it is equally important that all social workers (and not just psychiatric social workers) should keep up to date in their psychiatric knowledge. There must be no professional misunderstandings between psychiatrists and social workers because when these colleagues fail to understand each other's viewpoint it is the patient who suffers as a result.

We hope that you may have found reading this book a worthwhile exercise in communication.

Recommended Reading List

THE following list of titles for suggested further reading has been arranged according to the subjects of the chapters in the present work. This means that certain titles are mentioned more than once, but the arrangement means that the reader will more readily appreciate which book is recommended for a particular topic.

Chapter 1

G. CAPLAN (1961) *An Approach to Community Mental Health.* Tavistock Publications, London.

Chapter 2

A. BARNETT (1950) *The Human Species.* MacGibbon & Kee, London.
G. A. HARRISON and others (1964) *Human Biology.* Oxford University Press, London.
D. MORRIS (1967) *The Naked Ape.* Jonathan Cape, London.
D. ODLUM (1961) *Journey through Adolescence.* Penguin Books, England.
DAME E. YOUNGHUSBAND (1967) *Social Work and Social Values.* Allen & Unwin, London.

Chapter 3

D. B. BROMLEY (1966) *The Psychology of Human Ageing.* Penguin Books, England.
J. A. C. BROWN (1966) *Freud and the Post-Freudians.* Penguin Books, England.
R. FLETCHER (1966) *The Family and Marriage in Britain.* Penguin Books, England.
J. A. HADFIELD (1963) *Childhood and Adolescence.* Penguin Books, England.
J. H. KAHN (1965) *Human Growth and the Development of Personality.* Pergamon Press, Oxford.

Recommended Reading List

R. S. LAZARUS (1964) *Personality and Adjustment.* Prentice-Hall, New Jersey.

P. H. MUSSON (1965) *The Psychological Development of the Child.* Prentice-Hall, New Jersey.

J. & E. NEWSON (1965) *Patterns of Infant Care in an Urban Community.* Penguin Books, England.

D. ODLUM (1961) *Journey through Adolescence.* Penguin Books, England.

F. POST (1965) *The Clinical Psychiatry of Late Life.* Pergamon Press, Oxford.

D. W. WINNICOTT (1964) *The Child, the Family and the Outside World.* Penguin Books, England.

R. S. WOODWORTH (1965) *Contemporary Schools of Psychology.* Methuen, London.

WORLD HEALTH ORGANIZATION (1962) *Deprivation of Maternal Care—a Reassessment of its Effect.* W.H.O. Public Health Paper. No. 14. Geneva.

DAME E. YOUNGHUSBAND (1967) *Social Work and Social Values.* Allen & Unwin, London.

Chapter 4

E. W. ANDERSON and W. H. TRETHOWAN (1967) *Psychiatry,* 2nd ed. Baillière, Tindall & Cassell, London.

SIR D. HENDERSON and I. R. C. BATCHELOR (1962) *Henderson and Gillespie's Textbook of Psychiatry.* Oxford University Press, London.

Chapter 5

J. A. C. BROWN (1966) *Freud and the Post-Freudians.* Penguin Books, England.

E. E. IRVINE (1967) *Casework and Mental Illness.* Collected papers reprinted from the *British Journal of Psychiatric Social Work.* Association of Psychiatric Social Workers. London.

D. H. MALAN (1967) *A Study of Brief Psychotherapy.* Tavistock Publications, London.

C. RYCROFT (1966) *Psychoanalysis Observed.* Constable, London.

A. RYLE (1967) *Neurosis in the Ordinary Family.* Tavistock Publications, London.

E. J. THOMAS (1967) *Behaviour Science for Social Workers.* Free Press, Glencoe.

Chapter 6

M. CRAFT (1966) *Psychopathic Disorders.* Pergamon Publications, Oxford.

R. FOREN and R. BAILEY (1968) *Authority in Social Casework.* Pergamon Press, Oxford.

E. E. IRVINE (1967) *Casework and Mental Illness.* Collected papers reprinted from the *British Journal of Psychiatric Social Work.* Association of Psychiatric Social Workers, London.

DAME E. YOUNGHUSBAND (1967) *Social Work and Social Values.* Allen & Unwin, London.

Chapter 7

M. M. GLATT and others (1967) *The Drug Scene in Great Britain.* Edward Arnold, London.

N. KESSEL and H. WALTON (1965) *Alcoholism.* Penguin Books, England.

Chapter 8

N. W. FARBEROW and E. S. SHNEIDMAN (1961) *The Cry for Help.* McGraw-Hill, New York.

P. SAINSBURY (1955) *Suicide in London.* Chapman & Hall, London.

E. S. SHNEIDMAN and N. L. FARBEROW (1957) *Clues to Suicide.* McGraw-Hill, New York.

E. STENGEL (1964) *Suicide and Attempted Suicide.* Penguin Books, England.

Chapter 9

E. W. ANDERSON and W. H. TRETHOWAN (1967) *Psychiatry,* 2nd ed. Baillière, Tindall & Cassell, London.

A. COPPEN and A. WALK (1967) *Recent Developments in Schizophrenia.* Royal Medico-Psychological Association. Special Publication No. 1. Headley Bros., Kent.

A. COPPEN and A. WALK (1968) *Recent Developments in Affective Disorders.* Royal Medico-Psychological Association. Special Publication No. 2. Headley Bros., Kent.

SIR D. HENDERSON and I. R. C. BATCHELOR (1962) *Henderson and Gillespie's Textbook of Psychiatry.* Oxford University Press, London.

E. E. IRVINE (1967) *Case Work and Mental Illness.* Collected papers reprinted from the *British Journal of Psychiatric Social Work.* Association of Psychiatric Social Workers, London.

Recommended Reading List

Chapter 10

D. B. BROMLEY (1966) *The Psychology of Human Ageing.* Penguin Books, England.

F. FROST (1965) *The Clinical Psychiatry of Late Life.* Pergamon Press, Oxford.

J. HINTON (1967) *Dying.* Penguin Books, England.

P. TOWNSEND (1963) *The Family Life of Old People.* Penguin Books, England.

Chapter 11

G. CAPLAN (1961) *An Approach to Community Mental Health.* Tavistock Publications, London.

A. SAMUELS (1963) *Law for Social Workers.* Butterworths, London.

DAME E. YOUNGHUSBAND (1967) *Social Work and Social Values.* Allen & Unwin, London.

In addition, the following two short textbooks of psychiatry may be of help to the student: ·

F. J. FISH (1964) *An Outline of Psychiatry.* John Wright, Bristol.

M. SIM (1968) *Guide to Psychiatry*, 2nd ed. Livingstone, Edinburgh.

D. STAFFORD CLARK (1966) *Psychiatry for Students.* Allen & Unwin, London.

Index

Index

Coitus 16, 26, 150, 151
Cold, common 110
Colitis, ulcerative 109
Coma, insulin, in the treatment of schizophrenia 5
Communication, lack of, between doctors and social workers 13
Community
  mental disorder in the 9, 10, 78
  therapeutic *see* Environment, therapeutic
Compensation
  accident 99, 255
  psychological 28, 110
Complex 36
  inferiority 36
Conception 16, 27
Concussion 250
Conditioning therapy *see* Therapy, conditioning
Confabulation 167
Confidentiality 66, 160
Conflict
  oedipal 98
  psychological 48, 82
  psychosexual 125, 127
Conscience, lack of 136
Consciousness 32
Constipation, complaint of, in depression 207
Conversion, mechanism of 97
Convulsant drugs in the treatment of depression 5
Co-ordination, need for, in dealing with psychiatric illness 10, 11, 12, 13
Crime, sexual 140
Criminality 136, 137, 139, 142, 208
Crises, suicidal 191
Custody of mental patients 1, 2
Cycle, menstrual 16

Damage, brain 60, 120, 125, 144, 254
  during birth 18
Dangerous Drugs (Supply to Addicts) Act (1968) 183
DARWIN, CHARLES 30
Day Hospital 7
Daydreaming 49
Death 23
  gambling with 190
  instinct *see* Instinct, death
  modes of 186
Defence, manic 215

Defences, personality *see* Ego, defence mechanisms
Deficiency, vitamin 61, 166, 239
Delinquency 119, 120, 141
Delirium 55, 56, 166, 249 ff, 254, 257
Delirium tremens 166, 167, 251
Delusion 134, 167, 180, 207, 222, 244, 252
  primary 223
  secondary 223
Dementia 4, 55, 57, 59, 61, 97, 154, 167, 251 ff, 255
  pre-senile 259
Dementia praecox 219
Denial 33, 50
Dependence, drug 176
Depersonalization 95
Depression 51, 55, 84, 99, 116, 122, 123, 125, 126, 141, 150, 164, 189, 202, 248, 255
  causative factors in 209 ff
  endogenous 204 ff
  involutional 204
  neurotic 54, 85 ff, 203, 240
  psychotic *see* Depression, endogenous
  reactive 86, 203
  treatment of 213 ff
Depressive reaction *see* Reaction, depressive
Deprivation, emotional 45, 129, 135, 142
Development, physical 14 ff
Diagnosis, psychiatric 63
Dipsomania 168
Disease
  coronary artery 109
  skin 110
Disorder
  affective 55, 200, 202
  behaviour 50
  emotional 3
  personality 50, 55, 118 ff
  psychosexual 55, 135, 140, 146 ff
  sexual 51
Disorientation 167
Displacement 35
Dissociation 97, 129
Division, cell 17, 20
Drive, sexual 147
Drugs
  analgesic 176
  anticonvulsant 5, 256, 258
  antidepressant 88, 92, 107, 123

278

Index

Hospitals, general, psychiatric units in 6
Hostility in the informant 67
Hypertension 109, 243, 259
Hypnosis 85, 96, 108
Hypochondriasis 88, 90, 122, 126, 133, 135, 141, 205, 207, 241, 255
Hypomania 202, 203, 217
Hypothalamus 111, 112
Hypothermia 239
Hysteria 54, 60, 96 ff, 114, 121, 126, 128, 130

Id 32
Ideas, flight of 215
Identification 35
Illness
  depressive, constitutional factors in 60
  infectious 109
  physical, emotional factors in 11
  psychiatric, aetiological factors in 57 ff
  psychiatric, assessment of 52 ff
Immaturity 97
Immigrants 62
Impotence, sexual 147, 149 ff, 168
Impregnation, fear of 115
Incest 44
Individual psychology see Psychology, individual
Inebriation see Drunkenness
Infant
  newborn 19
  premature 18
Infantile sexuality see Sexuality, infantile
Inferiority 37
  complex see Complex, inferiority
Inferiority, organ 37, 110
Informants in history making 69
Injury, head 254
Inmates of hospital, chronic 2
Insanity 3
Insomnia 167, 241
Instinct 31
  death 34
  sexual 31
Institutionalization 2, 7
Insulin coma treatment 5
Intellect 46 ff
Intelligence, tests of 47
Intent, suicidal 187, 190
Interpersonal relationships see Relationships, interpersonal

Interpersonal Theory (of H. S. SULLIVAN) 37
Intoxication
  drug 178
  pathological 168
Intraversion 36
Isolation, social 239, 240, 249

Jaundice 182, 212, 250
Jealousy, pathological 168
JUNG, C. G. 36

KAY, D. W. K. see ROTH, M. and KAY, D. W. K.
Kibbutz 43
Korsakow's state 167
KRAEPELIN, EMIL 3

Latency period, the 39
Lesbianism 151, 156
Leucotomy, pre-frontal 93
Litigiousness 133
L.S.D. 108, 181, 226, 228
Lying, pathological 128, 137
Lysergic acid diethylamide see L.S.D.

Madhouses 2
Malaria in the treatment of syphilis 5
Maldevelopment, physical 28
Malingering 11, 99
Malnutrition 182
Mania 202, 215
  treatment of 217
Manic-depressive illness 44, 204, 131, 235
Manipulative behaviour 97, 100, 128
Marijuana see Hashish
Masochism see Sado-masochism
Masturbation 40, 125, 147, 149 ff
Mating 26
Measles, German see Rubella
Membranes, foetal 17
Menarche 20
  earlier onset of 21
Menopausal symptoms see Symptoms, menopausal
Menopause 22, 41, 58, 113
Menstruation 16, 17
Mental disorders, legal definitions of 265

Index